And She Danced For The King
—Memoirs of a Rockette

To order additional copies, please contact us.
BookSurge, LLC
www.booksurge.com
1-866-308-6235
orders@booksurge.com

RO TRENT
VASELAAR

AND SHE DANCED FOR THE KING —MEMOIRS OF A ROCKETTE

Imprint Books
2003

And She Danced For The King
—Memoirs of a Rockette

READERS COMMENTS

Absolutely wonderful life story. I felt as if I was there with her in all the amazing locations and reliving her life with her. Great read. Couldn't put it down.
Wenda McKee
Exeter, Devon, England

When one reads this delightful and engaging bio of a dancer tripping throughout the world, you are provided a personal insight to actual history of the famous Rockettes and the interactions of World War II ...it's a must read !
Ed & Carolyn Smith
Brentwood, TN

With Peg Morrison Macherey, what you see is what you get! Peg has always lived life to its fullest, and to be counted as her friend has added so much to my life........
Corliss Fyfe Whitney, Rockette '45-'53
Rockville Center, NY

What a remarkable Lady!. Reading this book was like being back at the Radio City Music Hall again. I got into the Hall some time after she had left, but had the pleasure of meeting her at the 75th Anniversary in N.Y. Treat yourself to reading her story.
Sandy Deel, Rockette '42-'45
Brentwood, CA

This very well-written book is a compilation of letters and comments covering ten years of experience one cannot buy. Each one is unique. Reading this book has been like reliving those exciting times, and has been a big thrill, since it is about one of my sisters.

Elizabeth Morrison Conrad
Peachtree City, Georgia

Being a former Rockette, I sat back and experienced every phase of Peg's life. And what an exciting life she had! A most enjoyable read.

Barbara Vaughan McCabe, Rockette '45-'50
Deer Park, NY

Dedicated to
my grandmother, Florence Morrison, who saved the letters
and
my mother, Ruth Morrison Van Fleet, whose selflessness
helped launch the story.

AUTHOR'S NOTE

In January 1995, my husband and I embarked on a belated honeymoon—a Caribbean Cruise. We made a stop in Vero Beach, Florida, so I could introduce Dave to two of my mom's sisters. Mom had passed away almost two years before, and seeing my aunts, Peg and Mary, was like reconnecting with my mother.

I was amused and delighted to watch Peg, still a flirt at eighty-three, thoroughly captivate my new husband as she regaled us with wonderful stories of her career as a dancer in the 1930's...performing for the King and Queen of England... escaping Hitler...Broadway openings... As we left Vero Beach, Dave asked me, "Is anybody writing this stuff down? Her stories are fascinating. They should be preserved."

Getting Peg's stories down on paper became my first post-retirement project. Initially, the idea was to preserve them for the family. However, I soon became fascinated by a career that mirrored an exceptional era in show business. It seemed too good not to share.

I was equally captivated by this testimony to family values. Values that drove Peg to write home with such unfailing regularity. Values that guarded her moral integrity through all those years in a business notorious for collapsing moral integrity.

Letters written daily to her family throughout her ten-year career provide an extraordinary chronicle of a turbulent and interesting time. And, tell the story of a nice girl from Cleveland, Ohio who followed her dream.

Peg and I combed through many boxes of letters and memorabilia. She moved in and out of a time warp as she relived her captivating stories. I moved right along with her and in the process came to know, understand, and appreciate a great deal about my own heritage.

PROLOGUE

One month shy of her 89th birthday, Margaret "Peg" Morrison Macherey, sits with Haley, her apricot miniature poodle, curled up in her lap, facing her computer screen. Her daily e-mail exchange with her two living sisters, Betty in Georgia, and Mary in Massachusetts, brings them in closer contact than they've ever been in their adult lives. A one-hour workout on the treadmill completed and dinner planned, she's ready for this journey down memory lane.

The two of us have spent several days combing through a large moving-box filled with letters written to her family during her ten-year show business career. It's been a daunting task, but we now have 10 shoe boxes filled with letters which we've filed in chronological order. Together we read through hundreds of letters. I come to know this remarkable woman in a whole new way. Reliving the life of a dancer in the 30's is fascinating.

It's a gray, raw day, as Nashville can be in February, but Peg is miles away in her thoughts. She is, in fact, a nineteen-year-old, leggy blond, full of dreams and resolve, heading for New York.

Margaret "Peggy" Morrison, the second of four girls born to Tom and Florence Morrison, entered the world on March 22, 1911, in Cleveland, Ohio. She grew up to follow her childhood dreams, albeit with slight modification. As a youngster, Peggy dreamed of becoming a missionary. "Not to spread the word of God necessarily, but to go to all those exotic places," she remembered many years later. And to exotic places she did journey—Paris, London, Buenos Aires, Biarritz, St. Louis, Chicago, Montreal…. And it wasn't her faith that got her there, but her legs!

The year was 1930 and America was reeling from the Great Depression. Everywhere, people were out of work and hungry. Ill health had recently forced Peg's own father, Tom Morrison, to give up his job as luggage buyer for the May Company Department Stores in Cleveland, Ohio. Her mother, Florence, worked as a secretary at the Cleveland Public Library. And her older sister, Ruth, answered her family's plea to forego her scholarship at Huron College in South Dakota and return home to help support the family. Peg's younger sisters, Betty and Mary, were sixteen and fourteen respectively.

Peg dreamed of show business providing her the vehicle to help the family. Her first letter home was filled with excitement and optimism, a tone that would become her hallmark.

Wednesday Nov. 26, 1930 New York City

Gee oh gosh oh golly am I ever excited. I never before in all my life got the thrill I'm getting now out of this here city! At the present I am sitting in my "hotel room", which is luxuriously furnished, eating an apple I bought for a nickel to help the unemployed. [Street vendors earning pennies to feed their families were a common sight.]

Peg's memories from the vantage of almost 70 years later were at odds with the reality of life in 1930. Time does have a way of erasing the unpleasant and magnifying the pleasant.

"I went to New York to give myself a rest from dance lessons," she reflected in 1999.

"I waited tables at Schrafft's and worked there a couple of months. I made a *ton* of money in tips and went back home to continue dance lessons until I felt 'ready' for the big plunge! I felt so rich when I returned to Cleveland I bought the family a gorgeous console radio. We all sat in front of it in the living room, listening, like we watch TV today!"

The journey into Show Biz had begun. The 30's were a golden era in show business. Both night clubs and live theater offered great opportunity for talented dancers. Road shows traveled the country by train and "doing the town" was all the vogue.

"I really believed that if I had ballet shoes I would know how to dance...all it would take was the right shoes," she recalled.

When she was about eleven, Peg borrowed a pair of ballet shoes from her school friend, Lucille, whose father, Frank Cain, was mayor of Cleveland Heights, Ohio, where the Morrison family lived.

During her junior year at Cleveland Heights High School, Peg's reputation as a good baby-sitter provided an opportunity that changed her life. She was asked to stay with a woman recovering from surgery. This woman, as it turned out, was a dance teacher.

"While I was caring for her she told me if I brought in two other students, she'd give me lessons for free." Very soon, Peg began her first formal dance lessons.

"A month before the first recital, I came down with mumps, first one side and then the other. I was devastated... sure my dancing career was over."

As a sixteen year-old entering her senior year in 1927, Peg's parents told her she could, "either have nice clothes, like your sister Ruth had her senior year, or dance lessons, but you can't have both." The choice was easy. She took the lessons and ventured to downtown Cleveland, for "real" lessons, studying classical ballet under Sergei Popeloff. This twice-weekly, 30-minute journey downtown on the streetcar continued for three years.

During the final year with Popeloff, Peg auditioned for a local production of *Madame Butterfly*. Selected as one of the dancers, Peg was elated. "I was in show business." She was on her way!

LEARNING THE ROPES
1931

Early in 1931 Peg returned to Cleveland from her initial
venture to New York City. She worked for Greyhound
Bus Company along with her older sister, Ruth, and
continued her study under Popeloff. By late summer of '31 she
had "the bug" again, so back to New York she went with $50
she'd saved from her paychecks.

Monday Sept. 7. 1931 New York City

*I'm here and what a heaven it is. I just wish you
could see it too. The location of the Club* [Dancer's Club, a
hotel where dancers lived for $7 a week] *is just terribly
"exclusive"... Had a lovely trip down and no trouble
or anything. There is a new Fred Stone show (Shubert
Theater) that is to soon start rehearsing so hope it isn't all
full yet. Say your prayers like you ner said 'em 'fore!'*

With just $50 in her pocket, Peg had to be frugal until
a real job came along. She allotted a dollar a day for food,
ten cents of which went for a cream cheese sandwich at
the Automat, a popular choice for economical food. Freshly
prepared food items were placed in individual, glass-front
compartments. A coin(s) placed in a slot would open the door
so you could retrieve your sandwich, salad, pie...whatever.
Automats were a mainstay of life in New York City until they
disappeared in the 1970's.

Watching her money was essential to Peg's survival. She toiled willingly to ensure her break would come. Understanding that her best potential was in tap instead of ballet, she worked hard to perfect her craft.

Thursday night Sept. 10

Talk about workouts! Billy Pierce, Wilma's tap teacher, whom she comes to every summer, thinks he has a "find" in me! He likes me just immensely and gave me an audition for this act. Well, I did my routines, but they were lousy! Absolutely terrible. I got all my taps in and did them the way I was taught but it was just not modern tapping. Outside of that the man and Billy Pierce were crazy about me—my figure, limbs especially!, face, smile and all that hooey—personality, etc. Well, Billy was so elated that he put me right to work in a private lesson on decent taps. That was about 3 PM yest'y. I had a private confab with him first and told him I guessed I was just out of luck because paying for lessons was just simply impossible and out of the question. I told him I had barely enough to live on. "Forget finances," he said. "And don't be afraid to eat plenty because you are coming in here at 11 or so and you're going to study and practice all day long for about a wk." By that time he hopes to get me ready for this act.

Since he likes me I think I am sure to get something good. And the best part is, he's giving me the training. He said I was a "high class" girl and I should NEVER accept a "cheap" job. I have class that 99% do not have.

With all those hours I practice, I eat like a horse, but cheap. Since yesterday I lost 2 lbs, but that only makes me 127, so don't worry. I tell everyone here I weigh 122! You can bet your boots I don't get on that scales in front of anyone of 'ems!

Hard work paid off quickly. Peg's first audition was for *Three's a Crowd*. The pre-Broadway tryout opened in New Haven on Oct. 14, 1931. The show had finished its Broadway run and was now going on the road, starring Fred Allen, Clifton Webb, Libby Holeman and Tamara Geva. Peg made the chorus line and worked under Albetina Rasch, the Austrian-born choreographer. Rasch, whose credits included Broadway musicals, Ziegfeld Follies and Hollywood films, is credited with incorporating classical ballet techniques into precision dancing, popular at the time.

Rehearsals were long and tough, but there was an air of excitement and anticipation. Preparing for the show's opening was grueling—good training for the years to come.

Monday, Sept. 21

I know you're anxious to hear about the first day of rehearsals. We started at 11 AM and first of all we had a vocal lesson. Yes, we sing songs and speak pieces and everything! After we did that for awhile, learned the tunes and some of the words, we started on the dances. The first one was the "Snake Hip" routine, which comes in the 2nd act and costumes for it are accordion pleated fancy pajamas. They call it the "sex" dance! Imagine! When I have to do those loose, double-jointed hips I can, I guess, as I got along pretty good. She had me in the front. We learned the entire routine and we were dismissed about 5:15. That was a lot earlier than I thought we'd get out. There are a million back bends in it, and it is the most strenuous dance I ever did! I'm so sore tonight I can hardly walk or bend.

Wednesday night, Sept. 23

It's after midnight I guess by now. I've lost all track of time. But I just had to let you know this tonight. Katherine [Peg's roommate at the time] *and I were both selected right off when all the girls had to dance for Madame Rasch. Of course, we haven't signed contracts or anything like that but I think we're pretty sure now. All we have to do is keep up the hard work and keep smiling for them.*

Friday night, Sept. 25

Well today was our 5th day rehearsing. Starting Monday we rehearse morning, afternoon, evening and night. Jerry, our stage mgr., said we may be working even as late as 1 or 2 AM! Sure glad Katheryn & I can stick together & we'll both have the other one to walk home with! Thank heavens, today now, we are almost all over our stiffness, and we can even walk downstairs and sit down, etc. Really, I thought we NEVER would live to tell the tale!

It won't be long until I'm home again—for a week, when the show plays Cleveland. And in the meantime I'll try and send you $10 a wk.

By the way, I have to pay that agent who sent me to this job $5 a week (10%) for 10 wks. Equal to 1 wk. salary. So for a while I'll be making $45. The first 2 weeks they take out Equity dues which amounts to $6 a wk ($13 a yr for dues). You have to belong to get a job, or you don't stay in. So Lord I hope I can get some home! I'll send the $12 you all sent me a different time.

PS Don't know if I thanked you or Ruth for the $1 you each sent but boy they looked like a million when I saw them. Thanks so much. I'll be doing that & more in a while for you all—

Financial assistance to the family was a common result of the economic hardships of the 30's, and the Morrison family was no exception. Peg's sister Ruth and their mother, provided the bulk of the family's support. Peg wanted, and was expected, to do her part as well. The erratic nature of show business made regular assistance to the family an on-going challenge, a challenge that persisted throughout her career.

Sunday, Sept. 27

Now we are SURE of our job. Isn't it too thrilling? Just think of it. And we open 2 wks from tomorrow. It seems really too good to be true but it is *true, and that's the unbelievable part!*

We have a day off rehearsal today, so Katherine & I had breakfast in the Club dining room. They have a radio in it and the room is as big as a minute. The room seats only 9 people and it's lit with candles. Just adorable. Well, it was the first I'd heard a radio since I left home and gee, the organ, and then a piano like Gene & Glenn, and then they played "Trees" and did I get blue? First time I think I was ever homesick.

We had costumes fitted this AM—practiced like mad until 2:30 and 3:30 again at Rasch's studio. Boy how they work us. We have 4 complete routines. The last one we learned last night and today. It's the "King's Horses" but they don't use that music any more, they use another piece just as cute. But oh! the number! It's all jumps and hops.

You ask about Madam R[asch]. *Well, she is Hungarian,* [actually, she was Viennese] *fat, short, very slick black hair, distinctive and* so far *adorable. She seems to like me although she doesn't know who I am from Adam, but she put me back into the first row as I told you about.*

In those days, dancers received no pay until after the show opened. All rehearsal time was without pay. Peggy had been in New York almost one month now and that original $50 was running precariously low. It was still two weeks until *Three's a Crowd* opened.

Thursday, Oct. 1

You say you are glad I'm eating enough. Well, it is a necessary evil and I've tried so hard to manage on what I brought. But the news is sad. I have another rent of $8 to pay, and live besides. I just counted my money and I have exactly $16.28 left. That's not so hot. It takes about $1.25 to 1.40 or .50 a day for me to live on now during rehearsals. Isn't that terrible? We try and do on less and it can't be done. Then of course I'll have to live a week in New Haven till I get some pay. I hate to think of asking you to send me any money, but if you can't do it I'll take Mr. AE Robinson [her great-uncle] *up on what he said, although I'd hate to do it. He said I shouldn't be afraid to ask him for some, but I assured him I wouldn't need any. If you couldn't, do you suppose Ruth could lend me some? As soon as I get to working I could send it right back. Let me know about it.*

Money was a constant source of anguish for everyone at this time. In a special delivery letter sent to her mother at work she presents yet another challenge.

Saturday, Oct. 3

Jerry and Ben Boyer talked to all of us today. They asked who of the girls had trunks. I, of course, raised my hand. But when they found out it was a flat one, they said I could use it if I wanted, but it was just their advice to get

*a wardrobe. Because you'd spend as much or more in cash &
in time for pressing and inconvenience. All those who don't
have any are urged to purchase. So Katheryn & I went to
the theatrical trunk store of NYC where* all *show people get
their trunks. It is the H & M Trunk Co. Daddy probably
knows of it. Well, what do you think I found? A second
hand,* clean *and repaired completely, H&M Trunk– ¾
size for $10! He had 6 people stand and jump on it and
guarantees it for 15 years....*

*But of course there's the money question. I have $5
left for food now that I paid my rent for the next wk. That
won't last me long. Please send me an answer about the
trunk & money* special air *mail pronto. I am embarrassed
to death about my money running out, but I swear I never
managed so skimpingly in all my life!...*

*Tell Daddy not to worry, that after I get on the road
& am earning my salary of $50 or $60 a week I'll buy his
medicine and he can tell Dr. Taylor to go to and stay put!*

So, Peg wrote her Uncle Horace's father, A.E. Robinson,
asking for a $20 loan, which she promised to repay as soon as
the show opened. He wired her $50 right away and told her
it was his contribution to her career, not a loan! "One of the
things I did with that money was go buy myself some black
underwear. Looking at all those goodies in the shop windows
along Broadway had gotten to me!!" she remembered over 60
years later.

Saturday night, Oct. 10

*I wrote Mr. AE and as soon as he rec'd it he wired
me money. So I am set 'till first salary pops up. We signed
contracts yesterday and get $50 a wk. Isn't that grand?*

And I hear that it is practically set that we're having a run in Los Angeles and all western cities! This is such a happy weekend.

With the opening just hours away, Peg reported to her family about the journey and the anticipation surrounding the biggest event yet in this young woman's life.

Tuesday Afternoon, Oct 13

Well, we're here. Our train left NYC at 11 this AM and the show had a special car. Some of the "Collegians" [show band] had a victrola and did we ever have fun. Gee—I got the biggest thrill pulling out of the Grand Central. New Haven is an awfully pretty town and so much bigger than I thot [sic] it'd be. We got in at 10 to 1 and immediately came here to the rooming house...The room we have is supposed to be $10 a wk, but we talked her down to $8 for the 5 nights. That's $4 a piece. Isn't that dickering for you? Must be getting to rehearsal. Thurs, (oh how I long for that day!) I'll tell you how we survived the opening night! I'll have you know there are absolutely mobs of people getting tickets at the box office. Whew! I'm thrilled already.

Wednesday, Oct. 14

Last night K [Katheryn] and I went through every single dance without a mistake. (Lord knows how!) We'll probably make ours tonight. But half the kids forgot everything last night. Two girls fell flat and cried their eyes out about it! But that means a wonderful performance tonight, Godfrey—we should have a MARVELOUS one!

Will write tomorrow and tell you about our first performance. Pray for us.

Three's A Crowd had a long run on the road. One of the members of the show band "The Collegians" was Fred McMurray, who later starred in many movies and the 70's sitcom, *"My Three Sons."* "In one of the skits, I had to hide behind a tree with him. Of course, that was before he was THE Fred McMurray," Peg recollected.

Life on the road was a new experience for Peg and her roommate, Katheryn. This was a time when family values and morals stood for something…even in show business. It was possible for "nice" girls to be successful, but they had to keep their guard up.

Sunday, Oct. 18 Newark

I'm kind of glad we're out of New Haven. The shows went OK but after each one you had to argue and fight your way when you left the stage door. Those Yale boys are kind of hard to convince that you don't care for their company. Boys! What we didn't say to some of them when they'd tag us! It's marvelous experience in how to take care of yourself! They won their game yest'dy from Chicago—27-0 and were they celebrating last night! Drinking right out of the bottle, right out on the street! *K* [Katheryn] *was scared skinny!*

Peg was off on a whirlwind with nightly performances, some matinees, and rehearsals in between. After Newark they played Washington, DC, Baltimore, Philadelphia, Pittsburgh and Cincinnati, followed by a wonderful Cleveland homecoming. Though the train was the preferred mode of transportation in the 30's, much of it was new to Peg. Up until now her only ventures beyond Cleveland had been by bus.

Wednesday night, Oct. 21 Newark

We leave here Saturday night after the show and take the Pullman to Washington, DC arriving there at 8 AM. My first ride! Hope my etiquette won't look too beginnerish! Katheryn's never been on one either.

Dating games show lots of similarities from generation to generation. Only the lingo changes as evidenced from this quick note from Washington, DC.

Oct 22, Thursday night.

Could have had an adorable date tonight but decided I'd squelch him and see how he took it. He's my partner in "Open Air" and darling. Said to me in the course of conversation, "How would you like to go out on a date tonight?" And I said, "With a prune—or a peach?" He said, "A peach of course." So I didn't know what to say! Finally I said, "But you all serve cream with the peaches, and I don't take cream!" How's that? So he said nothing more about the date!

The following day, Peg sent this further explanation.

About dates. Gee, we won't date married people so you might as well squelch them right off the bat. We've had dates practically every night this wk. Even had a date today that ended now—at 6:30—time to get ready for the show. We got breakfast & dinner out of it, and all the sights in Wash.

After the show tonight we have different dates from

*today's. They are peachy fellows and don't hound you or
coax you to if you don't drink or smoke. Of course, no matter
who we go out with, good fellows or otherwise (hardly
otherwise) we always are careful, naturally.*

For all the fun they were having, Peg anguished about
finances. She and Katheryn were continually cutting corners,
skipping meals, doing whatever they could to save money for
that "rainy day" when the show closed, as well as send money
home. Katheryn was the only one working in her family. On
several occasions, their pay from the show was cut by $10 if the
crowds had been lighter than expected. The country, after all,
was in the midst of "The Great Depression."

Sunday, Nov. 22 on the train to Pittsburgh

*In about 15 more minutes I'm going to have my first
dinner on a train. I can't wait. They soak you like the
devil, of course, but it's a necessary evil to eat and am I
starved.*

*Time has passed now and it's about 3 PM. Had my
dinner & it set me back exactly $1.70 including 15 cents
tip. Isn't that* terrible.

Life on the road, glamorous as it was, meant being away
from family on holidays.

Thursday, Nov. 26 Pittsburgh

*I'd planned on calling you for so long and then it was
all over so quick—gee, and was I ever thrilled? What did
you think when the operator said Pittsburgh calling? I was
so excited I couldn't wait while she was getting the number.
Did Ruth remember that I told her I was going to call? Or
maybe she didn't believe me.*

We've done 4 shows in 2 days and we're plenty worn out. Had a double-decker sandwich for Thanksgiving dinner. Couldn't eat turkey and then dance!

The second week of December the show played Cleveland. Sadly, no clippings survive, but her sister, Betty, who was seventeen at the time, remembers, "What a thrill it was for Peg to get some publicity for being a home town celebrity. She told me not to wave at her, and since we all [Mom, Dad and the three sisters] sat right down in front, that's exactly what I did—completely forgetting her admonition."

From Cleveland it was on to Detroit. The following special delivery went to her mother at work.

Tuesday, Dec. 15

Write special del what size glove Ruth [Peg's older sister] wears. I'm getting her pale blue long evening gloves for her formal.

Shortly before Christmas the show opened in Chicago's Erlanger Theater for a lengthy run.

Sunday afternoon, Dec. 20, Chicago

Here we are—believe it or not...Tell Mary [her 15-year-old sister] I'd be thrilled to death for her to come. I'd like to have Betty too, but I couldn't possibly afford to have 2 come. But Betty can have the next trip. Could Mary start Saturday AM, or sooner if you'd let her, so she'd get here by night? I could meet her after the show if she could get a bus coming in around 11 or 11:30 PM. I just can't wait. She'll be thrilled to death with the city, but before she leaves, make her promise to go back. She's liable to want to stay!

By the way, is Ruth's Bill coming to Chicago to keep his date with me? Tell him to call me here. I'm counting on Xmas dinner with him! And I've Amily Ideal, the German girl in the show, anxious to meet him so she can converse with him in her native tongue.

At the time, Ruth was dating a German student, Bill Plambeck, studying at Case Institute in Cleveland.

Monday night, Dec. 21

The package arrived & I went after it. Of course I had to open it and find out what the "Live" was in it. Well, were we tickled! Gee it is darling. *Got it home and put all the trimmings on it & it looks too adorable for words. The rest is just burning me up. I'm having someone keep my stuff for me till Xmas Eve. Packages from Robinsons arrived today.* [Peg's Florida relatives who had sent her the $50 "contribution to her career"] *Yours and theirs will be all I'm getting. But that's enough all right & it'll be a wonderful Xmas even though there isn't $$$ flying around!*

Be sure to send Mary as SOON as possible. We just can't wait for her to come. Send her for Xmas if you can and want to.

Wednesday aft., Dec. 23

Yesterday I was walking home up Michigan Ave—it's about 10 blocks. All the way you could hear organ music playing Xmas songs and gee it was the most impressive thing.

The Chicago run of *Three's a Crowd* was a favorite holiday event. The show played to packed houses against stiff competition.

Saturday night between shows Dec. 26

The show could last about 8 or 10 weeks here then maybe to the west coast. Last night Jolson opened and there wasn't a single seat vacant in our *house. Nor this afternoon either. We're so successful here. Why if this keeps up we may be getting full salary starting next week!*

I've been thinking of Mary all day—on her first long trip. The whole company is awaiting her arrival. I called the station and they're going to send someone over with her in a cab. The bus gets in at 8:50. Gee I can't wait. I wish she or one of you could come and stay forever. *I'm so lonesome right now. Mom, you know when I talked to you and Daddy I was so thrilled and kept the tears back, but when Ruth's voice came…You can't imagine how I love you all & her too. Golly, I just had to burst out. I'm so darned glad she can come over here too. I only wish you and Daddy & Betty could come too. Betty talked so well over the phone. I hope she could hear me. Could she??*

Must run and do the show now…and await the best Christmas package of all—that's coming by taxi to visit me.

Peg's sister, Betty, who was deaf, had recently started attending classes offered by the Association for the Hard Of Hearing where she learned to read lips and benefited from speech therapy. A chance to talk on the phone was a new experience for her.

Tuesday night, Dec. 29

The show is still going great. Packed *house all the time. We are in the papers all the time. "Best bet in town" etc. etc. We're pretty thrilled. Hope it keeps up awhile.*

***

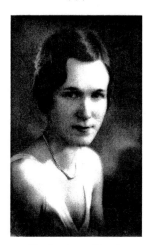

Peg's sister Ruth

LIFE ON THE ROAD
1932

The fortunes of show business often changed overnight. Sell-out one day, sparse audiences the next, reminded all that the Depression was still a reality. The New Year dawned with renewed uncertainty about the show's future and continued struggles with money.

Wednesday night, Jan. 6 Chicago

We found out tonight that we'll run next week anyhow. We've "heard" we will play here till the 23rd—that's 2 more weeks. We go back to our cut salary—40 bucks—this Sat. Isn't that the limit? It's to cut expenses more. Collegians have taken about a 45% cut, and the 3 stars will play for expenses only. So you see they're doing everything in their power to keep going. It burns us up—the cut again—but what can one do. Imagine! One week back [to full salary] & cut again. You should have seen the mass meeting we all had, but there's just nothing to do but take it. It's better than nothing. I only hope we go to the coast.

Later the same day

From the audience the last 2 nights it looks like business is dropping down somewhat. And things look suspiciously as if this "West Coast" talk was a lot a hooey. We'll know by tomorrow night if we close this Saturday.

The uncertainty about the show's future dragged on. One day they planned for an extended run that would put them on the West Coast through spring...the next day closing was imminent. The cast kept its spirits up, finding fun in rubbing elbows with famous stars of the day.

Thurs., Jan. 14

Last night who do you think sat in the front row— right plum in front of me? Eddie Cantor & George Jessel [popular comedians] *and their wives. Gee were we thrilled. Between the acts they were back stage and we saw them. And they were at the party last night that we were at. Cantor's a scream.*

Later that week the show moved to St. Louis, opening on Sunday, January 24. Through the continuing uncertainty about the show's future, Peg worked hard to keep her spirits up, or at least to keep them up in her letters, so as to not upset the family back in Cleveland. The bomb came.

Friday, January 29

Prepare yourself now for the worst. Notice hasn't gone up yet but all things look like we go no further than Kansas City next week. We will know definitely next Monday & I shall write a special del. [delivery] *and let you know. There isn't any use worrying about it. I'll just have to save all this week's salary & next week's and that'll keep me a few weeks back in NY. We've had the lousiest crowds here imaginable, that's why.*

Address next week's mail for me to the Park bench— the softest one—I'm saving my dough!

Don't worry. I'm not. Everything happens for the best.

This unbridled optimism, a Morrison family trait, played a large role in Peg's show business success. Even today, she and her sisters frequently remind each other that "everything happens for the best."

Sunday evening, Jan. 31 Kansas City

This town is so funny. All the buildings are very low & it looks so hick townish but I imagine it's very nice in the residential sections. Just think, I'm exactly halfway across the continent. Well that's not so bad for the 1st job. Maybe the next one will take me further.

But the crowds improved in Kansas City and the show took on new life.

Monday night, Feb. 1

The list for next week went up tonight. We leave here Sunday morning and go to Des Moines where we play on Mon night. Then we leave there on Tues AM and Mother, we'll go right thru Cleveland I'm sure! We go to Rochester NY and travel all Tues and Tues night. I think we'll probably hit Cleve around 12 or 1 AM. That's Tues night. And gee I hope you can have the family down there. We'll stop I imagine—even if it's only for a few minutes.

We'll leave Rochester on Thurs night after the show and go to Springfield, Mass. where we play Fri night, Sat matinee & Sat night, then leave there Sun AM for Boston. We'll play there for 2 weeks!

Tonight's audience was unbelievably huge—and so

marvelous looking. Everyone in dress clothes and they're so appreciative, & get all the jokes. I'm surprised they get so many, being this far away from NY.

There is a Forum cafeteria here. Tonight my dinner was the huge sum of 25 cents!

The weeks and weeks of uncertainty about the show's future came to an end February 27 as the show closed in Boston. Youthful exuberance and healthy self-esteem enabled Peg to look to the future with excitement, seeing beyond the frightful economic conditions gripping the United States. It was as if show business were isolated from the country's woes.

Sunday night, Feb. 28

Well Mom, it's curtain time now, but no curtain's going up tonight. And I can truthfully say I'm glad. You know why? Because you don't get anywhere doing the same thing too long—right? Tomorrow starts another search for work. There's work to be had & if you look far enough for it I know darn well it's to be found. I'm really all excited. It's like another new adventure.

The next day she wrote her sister, Ruth...

The first day is over and plenty is accomplished. Honey, I'm so happy, I'm all a twitter & a twitch. I'm moving Wednesday to 150 W. 77th St. Phone is Susquehana 7-9124. We pay $6 each a week and we can save cooking in—live on $3 a week each, easily.

Went down to Billy Pierce and he said we (Helene & I) would be working in 2 weeks. He says he can't begin to tell me how much I've improved.

Good as his word, on March 18, three weeks after the show closed in Boston, Peg opened at the Paramount, in New York, just a few days shy of her 21st birthday. Of course her friends all thought they were celebrating her "19th." True to the custom in those days, she seldom divulged her real age. One of the stars in that show was Bob Hope. His entrance followed one of the dance numbers. Peg recalled the night he missed his cue, "We had to repeat our number and he came running out on stage, all out of breath. It got a lot of laughs."

Very soon they were back on the road...playing Buffalo, Detroit, Chicago, St, Louis...when in New York, Peg and her pals tried to take advantage of theater passes whenever they had the chance.

> *April 20, Wednesday night NY*
>
> *Tonight we saw "Hot Chicago" which just inspired me so that I feel now like I can go out and conquer the stage marvelously! Buddy Rodgers is so adorable, Bert Lahr too. Best of all, most sensational, is Eleanor Powell, who I saw in "Fine & Dandy." She's a tap dancer & in my mind the most marvelous dancer on the stage today. Words just don't describe her!*

The Morrison clan tried to catch Peg's show whenever she was anywhere close to Cleveland. In April 1932, her sister Ruth, surprised her in Buffalo and then joined the troupe on the train. Their visit provided time for planning and dreaming. Peg responded to a subsequent letter from her mom.

> *Thurs., May 12 Detroit,*
>
> *So Ruth told you I have "picture ambitions?" You bet I have. Between you and me and the gatepost. Mom, so many people have said I would be the good type—people*

who have worked in pictures & know. Here's what I'm going to do. Get into a NY (if possible) show and during the day, invest money in voice and speech training and see if I can get some little start. You must *have your voice trained & know a little something about acting. All that I'm going to prepare for. I get thrilled to think about it—it's something to work for. And pictures are really more profitable than shows. If you're good you get a* contract, *which means you get paid if you're working every day or not.*

Peg returned to New York in early summer and waitressed at Scharfts to put food on her own table and a roof over her head. She quit the job in late fall to rehearse for a new Broadway show, *April in Paris,* with Bea Lilley. The choreographer liked her dancing and had her front row center. This was still the era when it was possible to rehearse for two weeks before you got paid. At the end of the two weeks, Peg and two other dancers were bumped from the show. The producer had just returned from Europe and had to make room in the line for three of his girlfriends.

Almost 70 years later she remembered, "After I cried my eyes out for about two weeks, someone told me about a ballet audition. It called for sixteen arabesque releveés on toe! They were not my forté, but my guardian angel pulled me up sixteen times! I got the job, and we signed a contract for $27.50 a week at Paramount in Paris. I'd been getting $40-50 a week in *Three's a Crowd.* I was down to my last fifteen cents. I used five of it to make a collect call to Mother and Daddy to tell them, 'One week from today I'm sailing for Paris!' We got the $27.50 in advance, which was like a million dollars to me. We rehearsed all week and the following Friday, December 9, we sailed on the S/S Paris."

Peg's eyes welled-up with tears as she continued, "God was taking care of me. That's why I got kicked out of that show. Almost everything from then on developed because of that job in Paris."

Florence and Tom Morrison journeyed to NY to see their daughter off. Peg's beau, Joe Ancona, a saxophone player, accompanied them. Tom's health was deteriorating steadily, so this was quite a jaunt for him. It must have been a bittersweet parting as the three bid farewell to this young woman they all loved and sent her off on a greater adventure than any of them had ever dreamed.

The first day out Peg wrote the details to her sister, Ruth.

Saturday, Dec. 10

Honey I'm looped already on the wine from luncheon! A bottle of red wine & one of white wine is on each table and you drink that instead of water! And my dear, everything is served separately. First you get soup, then hors d'oeuvres...then a clean plate and fish & potatoes. Another clean plate & asparagus, another clean plate & a piece of steak, another clean plate & peas—another plate & cheese & crackers—another plate & salad & another with dessert. Then coffee (which is so strong it's thick) or tea. It takes about an hour to go thru all the courses. Oh yes, fruit comes after the cheese. It's a positive scream.

Well, now to tell you about last night. Mother, Dad & Joe came down. Got down to my cabin & there were a whole bunch of letters, all yours, & the card. There was a box of flowers. Beautiful baby chrysanthemums & a card saying, "When she pitches and rolls, hold everything—Auntie Marie, Uncle Horace & Marian." I was thrilled to tears.

*About 15 minutes later your flowers came from the office &
honey they were* gorgeous*! I never saw such a beautiful
array in my life. Gosh, it made me feel so marvelous to
think the kids were so thoughtful and so darling to think
of me and do such a glorious thing like that. Mom, Daddy
& Joe left about 20 to 6 & they didn't wait to see the boat
pull out. I'm just as glad because the "good bye" was over
all at once. Hope Daddy stands the trip back all right. It
was quite tedious for him coming down to the boat.*

*After dinner we had our cabins changed to 1st
class—about 6 times larger than the one Mom will describe
to you. When we return to the cabin the stewardess draws
your bath and you bathe in salt water & you simply can't
get a lather of soap. A panic.*

Friday am, early Dec. 16 Le Havre—at last

*I simply can't sleep. It's 3 AM and we are supposed
to be in bed at 1 AM…our boss's orders. We just now
came into Havre & it is gorgeous, all the lights at night.
I'm simply thrilled to pieces. I can only see it out of our
porthole. I can hear the people on deck singing all sorts
of songs—Hail, hail, the Gang's all here, etc. We docked
at Plymouth, England about two hrs to unload mail and
passengers, about 4 PM today. Talk about being glad to see
land after only water for 6 days and 7 nights!! OH BOY!
It was the most beautiful sight. The sun was just going
down and I'm telling you—against that beautiful green
shore, so quaint—and all the fishing boats in the harbor—
it looked like a painted picture. I wish you could have seen
it. I am thrilled now for the 1st time since we pulled out.
I was thrilled then, but I got so lonesome—honestly you*

couldn't' have any *idea how terrible I was. I'd swear I'd save $100 and break my contract and come home as soon as I saved enough for my passage! But, I guess anyone would get Gawd-awful ideas in their heads in the middle of the Atlantic Ocean!*

Last night they had a big floor show in 1st Class. We were the main attraction and we did a kick routine. The boat was rocking so we could hardly stand on our feet. Afterwards some big shot movie man gave us a big champagne party—ah deah!

The week before we left was like a dream. Suddenly in mid-ocean it became a terrible lonesome reality. Now, it is beginning to be a dream again.

Friday, Dec. 23 Hotel des Sylphes 5 Rue Lafayette, Paris

My first mail in 2 weeks! 11 letters for me. *I'm ecstatic!*

We opened yesterday & we do 2 dances in the show— 5 shows a day. Each show lasts 18 minutes and that is very long. Generally they last 12 min at the most. We were on stage in costume & make up at 7 AM, went through the show 3 complete times then *did our regular 5 shows!*

This strenuous work is doing wonders to me. My legs are getting so marvelously thin and I'm much thinner all over.

I'm doing right well by the French in my broken down and neglected French tongue. I can get what I want in restaurants, stores & the hotel—and I'm the "speaker" of our bunch of kids. More fun! It's just like we're in a new world. I love it here though, but do miss everyone terribly.

Tonight is Xmas eve and I can't imagine it. All us kids are having a champagne party (and port wine) with cheese and crackers and French pastry down in our room (we have the Xmas tree) and then tomorrow we are all having a real American dinner at the one American restaurant here. Imagine after 2 wks and more to have a good cup of coffee. I've been drinking tea & chocolate and don't waste my 2 francs on their gawd-awful coffee.

Tonight before the party we are going to midnight Mass at the Church of the Madeleine. They say it's just gorgeous. I've seen it from the outside.

That was the first, of what would be many Christmases for Peg, in a foreign land.

THE PRICE OF STARDOM
1933

A year that promised many new adventures dawned with the obvious comparisions to home.

Sunday, Jan. 1, 1933

Dearest Ruth,

New Year's Day in Paris, and instead of snow & cold we have a perfect spring day, blue sky and sun—for a wonder, cause it sure loves to rain here!

Did I tell you about this fellow I met on the boat, René, who is the son of a millionaire champagne maker here? [René Heidsieck of Piper Heidsieck Champagne] *He's sailing to NY again this week so Tues. night we're going on a farewell party to a snooty place called the Lido. Very formal. When you get there, the way I understand it, you find a very gorgeous dance floor, a marvelous orchestra & around the dance floor or at one end, is a swimming pool. So, you see people in gorgeous formal attire or in bathing suits. Isn't that fun?*

Last night 6 of us girls didn't have dates for New Year's Eve so we marched ourselves to the American Café des Artistes and there upon found gobs of Americans & we drank the New Year in with Champagne. We all had a grand time—got home at 3:30, and it cost us each 20 francs (80cents) for all the champagne & sandwiches and everything. Imagine!

We get the NY Herald every day & it seems it always has some Cleveland news in it.

The theater wasn't all glamour. It was lots of work…hard work.

Thursday, Jan. 5

We opened the new production today & it is more gorgeous & stupendous than a NY show. It's OUR show! We do everything in it & we are a huge success. Mr. Rasset was so thrilled with our performances that he couldn't get words to tell us. And yet, we DIE on our toes from that toe ballet filler we do. It sure is awful long & hard—about 14 choruses in all! Imagine. We were rehearsing till 2 AM last night, & had to be in makeup & on stage at 6:30 AM! I ask you! I'm simply dead.

Just took a grand hot bath & will flop back on my pillow now—to sleep.

Next mail comes tomorrow as a boat arrived today. Hope I get a lot!

Wednesday, Jan. 11

Next Monday night we are to dance for oh a whole bunch of kings and queens, and presidents & ambassadors, dukes, bishops, cardinals, Popes, etc from what we gather. We're doing the toe ballet from this show & also a little filler routine we just put together. We're to get about 10 francs extra pay for it (40cents)!! But it'll be grand to say "we've danced before so & so, and so & so, my deah!"

Mary's [Peg's 16-year old sister] *letter in French was great. I'll answer her in French as soon as I can find time.*

Peg and her roommate, Mary Brooks, spent their mornings taking French lessons. In another letter to Ruth, written the same day, she exuded excitement.

Wednesday, Jan. 11th

Honey I'm in heaven—ecstasy, in a trance. I'm going to COLLEGE. Doesn't that sound wonderful? To the Alliance Français, taking French every morning from 9-11 is the lesson & 11-12 is lecture. I simply am nuts about it, have learned so much. My roommate, Mary, goes with me. We have a terrible time getting out of bed it's so darned cold & dark and we're so tired.

Monday night we danced at the International Club for all these notables. Went over right after our last show, in limousines and what a gorgeous place. Ruth, it's just like a palace. You go in the drive & there is a huge court. Next you see some steps and lo & behold on either side of the steps there are guards or something, in gorgeous red & black uniforms, carrying gold swords & wearing gold hats.

We did our toe ballet & a little filler. Honey, if you could have only seen our stately, royal looking audience. We saw the list of guests and Ruth, talk about royalty… princes, princesses, counts, ambassadors, cardinals, & most important of all, the Pres. Of the French Republic, Pres. Albert Lebrune. It was so thrilling!

Peg also shared the success of those lessons in a letter to her sister, Betty.

Sunday, Jan. 15

Just had more fun writing Mary a letter in French. Hope she can understand it OK.

Wish you could have seen or been at that formal I went to last night. It was more fun. Ye gods, I never had so many men around me—I felt like a Cinderella! And my dear, I just chatted away in French. More fun. There were thousands of people there & it was a lovely sight, gorgeous gowns etc. It was at the Cuban University & everyone spoke either French or Spanish. Soooo I spoke French!

Saturday, Jan. 28

Last night we danced at a big swanky *hotel—the Hotel Majestic. It was all the biggest shots in the Paramount organization. We did last week's show, the toe dance, snake hip & fast jazz—all on a carpet & no stage, we were on the same level as the spectators. Who do you suppose sat right in front of where I was dancing, but Clara Bow [popular screen star] & Rex Bell. She sure looks different.*

The rigors of their schedule left little time for relaxation. Being so far from home, with communications erratic, since all mail traveled by ship, sometimes their morale flagged a bit. Peg poured her heart out to her Mother.

Wednesday, Feb. 15

Finally, we have a bit of time to breathe and take life easy for 8 hours. Ah me! Aren't they kind? But we love it. We're a bunch of G___damn fools to take it—by golly. I like to dance but believe me when you're worked as if you are some sort of machine & instead of filling you up with gas & oil to make you work, you are filled with swear words, threats etc, I call it inhumane!

For the past week they have rehearsed us until we

*were all hysterical & crying—even for the shows on stage.
It's a perfect fright. He [Rasset] doesn't think he can get
anything out of us unless he calls us "bitches, bastards, god
damned idiots, etc"! I'm actually beginning to think my 4
years of training hasn't done a darned bit of good. That I
was never meant to be a dancer. I might as well go scrub
floors and I think I'd be much more appreciated. God! I
don't mind working hard, but there's a difference between
that & being driven & worked like a slave or a dumb
animal with nothing in return. They got us to the theater,
on stage & in make up at 6 AM this morning & we hang
around for 1 hour, while they finish scenery etc. Of course
they couldn't call us for 7 or 7:30,but no, everything is
done so unsystematically & so bassackwards [sic] that lots
of times you think you're wrong!*

Those bouts of anger and frustration were short-lived
though. The sixteen-week contract at the Paramount ended
in late April. Mickey Rasset chose half of the girls from the
line to dance at the Casino in Biarritz. The rest were booked
into the Prince of Wales Theater in London. "By the time we
went to London," Peg remembered, "I was doing my thinking
and dreaming in French. At first, I felt awkward reverting to
English. For a few days, phrases like 'bread & butter' and 'come
in,' would only come to me in French!

"We met some young men in London who invited us to a
party. They'd stocked up on liquor and were blown away that
we didn't drink. Their impression of American girls was that
they drank *lots*!

"The job at Prince of Wales Theater was a steady line-
up, like we'd done at the Paramount. We'd been there about
a month when I got a cablegram from Mickey Rasset saying

that he had an opening for me in Biarritz. I was astounded and excited. I knew I couldn't get out of the London contract, so I just left. My buddies in the line covered for me...put their make-up on my stand so I wouldn't look gone until I could actually get out of town!

"As the train traveled through France, I had such a guilty conscience that when I saw the conductor, or at least he was a man in uniform, coming through the car looking at passports, I just *knew* they were after me! When my turn came, I gave him my passport, he looked at me...back at the passport...at something in his hand...back at me...for an agonizingly long time. Finally he handed my passport back, said '*merci*' and was on his way. I was so relieved I wasn't about to ask what he was looking for!"

When Peg arrived in Biarritz, she rehearsed long and hard to learn the numbers. Rasset was a stern task master. Your best wasn't good enough for him; he expected more. The girls did two shows a night...one at 12:30 AM and one at 3 AM. This was, after all, a casino.

"We'd go to bed about six in the evening and sleep until about 10:30 or 11, then go do our makeup and get ready for the shows. One night about 10 PM," Peg recalled, "We were awakened and told we had to do an early show. One of the gals sputtered, 'Geez, the way they're acting you'd think the Prince of Wales was here!' Guess what? It was the Prince of Wales and Wallis Simpson, (who later became the Duke and Duchess of Windsor). We all danced right to him."

When the job in Biarritz ended late that summer Peg went back up to Paris where she landed a job at the Folies Bergère doing classical ballet, a real change from the steady line-up. While in rehearsals for the Folies, she also took a job with an English troupe, the Bluebelle Girls, at the Moulin Rouge in Montmartre, to earn some extra money. The kind of tap dancing they did was quite different from American tap. It was a real challenge, and exhausting. "I was a zombie," she reminisces. "Working at Moulin Rouge, Folies rehearsals often overlapped. One dress rehearsal...wherever we were, there were these big pipes...I curled up on one and went sound asleep!"

***

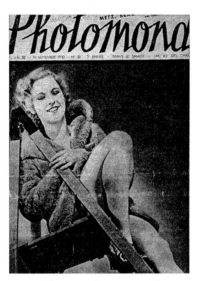

Photomonde cover girl
23 September 1933

***

Even the grueling schedule allowed time for some fun. Peg and her American friends became acquainted with three young Frenchmen, René Calderon, Roger Sasso and Hubert Beauveux, known to his friends as Cupid. The young men were only too happy to show their city and some of the countryside to the three American dancers. When time permitted, the six of them enjoyed the sites around Paris, even took off for the beach at Deauville, on occasion. The friendships became an important part of Peg's life.

Traditional American holidays still called for traditional celebrations, though.

Thursday—Thanksgiving [Nov. 23]

Got up at 4:30 (PM) today and went to the Chicago (an American Restaurant) for Thanksgiving dinner. Everything from soup to nuts. My lordy I could hardly fasten my costumes tonight. Went through the show with no stops whatsoever tonight & it went rather well—except yours truly missed 2 numbers—one being my "big part" modeling the gown. It's a long wait and they should ring me, so when I didn't get a ring for so long I went down & they screamed *at me and boy I screamed back! I've hung around down there night after night & my feet are so sore—we have 11 pair of shoes to break in. And believe me they can exercise their finger and press the button to ring for me! Boy was I furious.*

The other one I missed is a perfectly impossible change. The idiotic dresser we have puts all 16 costumes in a pile *& the shoes & hats as well & nothing was sorted. That dresser is more bother than a help!*

Well, tomorrow night we actually open *. Believe it or not, after 11 weeks of rehearsing. The show is still a mess & I pity the poor people tomorrow night when it comes to some of our dances. They've been changed and riddled to death at the last moment until no one knows what they're doing. I'm not excited about the opening night cause I'm too tired. We've rehearsed till dawn every night.*

Monday, Nov. 27 Paris

For the first time we did the entire *show* [Folies] *in costume, scenery & orchestra. Before we've taken one act a night. Oh Mom, I'd give anything for you to see this show. The costumes are simply the last word. You know, since I seem to be a big favorite of Mistinguett* [the star of the Folies] *I am always having costumes completely different from the other girls. It's more fun. And that evening gown that I model—well all the kids say it's the most stunning of all the ones shown. It's pale green. My hair is so very blonde that it just looks great. I've never been so thrilled with anything in my life.*

My next biggest thrill is being up front with all the "artistes" (stars) in the grand finale. The costumes are beautiful. Gee I'm so thrilled. Mistinguett is adorable to me. Boy, I am sure glad I'm at the Folies and not a back line stooge with the other girls at the Casino.

Well, Mom, the costumes & scenery for this show must have cost millions. Everything is in the best of velvets, furs, silks and satins. Back drops of sequins—and exquisite scenery. One number is of snowmen. The costumes are all from head to toe, white fur! They're marvelous.

And Mistinguett is perfect. What a sense of humor! And even at her age she's simply adorable on stage. Talk about a personality! [Her age at this time was rumored to be 67, though she was actually 58, and, purportedly, her legs were insured for $1 million.]

Can't think of any more news. It's daylight now. Better get some sleep. We've been going since 4 PM to 6 AM! Do write soon.

Friday, Dec. 1

We opened tonight at last. Everything went perfectly...it was such a thrill. I just danced my fool head off and did so enjoy it. Mistinguett's entrance was simply—superbly—the last word. The whole stage is in pale pink & pink ostrich feathers. There are steps of silver and at the top a cage all covered in shades of pink feathers. After much movement of people, the "Spark Ballet" (I'm in this with the principals), the doors to the cage open and its all rhinestones inside & there is Mistinguett. She descends the stairs & she's dressed in a gorgeous blue dress studded with rhinestones, has a rhinestone little hat on her head with blue feather—and wears a blue feather boa about 10 yards long. Well, they clapped and roared and whistled and cheered and clapped for 5 or 10 minutes—it seemed years. Finally she could begin to sing—an adorable song about herself. And they'd clap and applaud & cheer in the middle of it. What a thrill! I was so thrilled I felt like crying. It just gives me goose pimples to think about it.

Well, it's 4 AM and I must get to bed. Oh, Mom, I'm furious. The one time I get my name in the program for something special I'll have you know they've put me as "Phyllis Morison." Can't even spell Morrison right, let alone Peggy!

Mistinguett, "Queen of the Paris Music Hall," was born Jeanne Bourgeoise in 1875. She became the most popular French entertainer of her time, of the Garbo & Dietrich genre. As Maurice Chevalier described her, "She had a way of moving which was the pinnacle of grace, but she was more than loveliness alone—she was Paris, the symbol of gaiety and good humor and courage and heart."

More than 66 years later Peg relived that 1933 opening. "Mistinguett was the STAR at the Folies. She'd been there forever. When she made that entrance, adorned all in blue, she hypnotized me with her stare. She locked her gaze on me from the top of the steps all the way down. All the dancers were below with arms up toward her and she locked onto my eyes and held them all the way down."

As she approached her second Christmas in Paris, Peg began to feel the vastness that existed between herself and the rest of her family back in Cleveland. At the same time Mistinguett continued her effort to cast her spell over Peggy Morrison. "I began to realize that she had her eye on me in a way that made me really uncomfortable," Peg reflected. She began to talk about going home.

Thursday, Dec. 14

Well, I guess I've made up my mind. Mistinguett or no Mistinguett, I'm going home & I think I'll leave in Jan.

Friday, Dec. 15

Tonight we had a big party to celebrate 1 year since we arrived—it's a year today. What I liked about this party was that you didn't have to drink. I mean this—nobody tagged after you and kept insisting that you join in & making you do nothing but argue all night! It was lovely.

I still have not changed my mind about going home. I think I'll be sailing about Jan. 31—maybe even Jan. 17—I don't know for sure yet.

Monday, Dec. 18

One wk from today is Xmas—think of it. You think of it, it makes me sick when I do!

You know I told you I had an idea Mistinguett would make advances? Well, for 3 nights in a row now she's done something that gives me the willies. In the Jardin de Neige scene we do a dance & then finish in a diagonal leading from the steps when Miss. makes her entrance. As she comes down those steps for the past 3 nights she has stared that intense stare right into my eyes so that I can not for all I'm worth, get my eyes off hers. You know that hypnotic glare! It just scares me to death. Then last night I got the blues something awful & I was tired anyhow. I was waiting for my mannequin part and was sitting in a little dark room right off the boxes and for no reason I started to cry. Miss's little blond sec'y came by and must have seen a tear glistening on my cheek. So she put her arm around me and asked what was the matter. I said I was tired, that was all. So she kissed me on the cheek and said if I had any troubles or heartaches just to come & tell them to her & Miss. She felt so badly because I was crying. Really she was adorable, but can you see where that hitches up?? I sure can! Maybe it's a good thing I decided to come home in Jan.

If Miss. makes advances she'll no doubt offer me stardom, but I'd prefer marriage to stardom gotten that way! She's powerful & wealthy & famous & all that, & she can do everything she wants, but if she "wants" me I'm afraid she'll get stung this once, no matter what her pay is. She and her darling little sec'y have been so darned sweet to me. I've spent plenty of time in her gorgeous dressing room eating bon-bons & listening to her radio, etc and they've been perfectly charming so far. But I guess I shan't accept anymore candies now.

Peg was tired, very homesick, continued to have financial struggles and she was ridiculed by many of the dancers because of the special recognition she was getting. Those things, along with growing apprehension about just why she was getting all this attention from Mistinguett, were wearing on her.

Wednesday, Dec. 20

Did I tell you I dreamt I was home the other night. I surprised everyone. Walked in the front door & Daddy was listening to the radio. I kissed him & told him to be quiet I was going to surprise everyone. So I went into the kitchen & you were in there with so many people. I remember distinctly seeing Auntie Clyde. Without even saying hello to me or anything, you told Ruth to get a pencil & paper & sit me down to figure out where my money went when I was working here (Europe). And I sat down with her & gave her Marguerites's [Peg's roommate] *& my budget. Then I got furious & decided since it was 2 days before Xmas I'd still have time to get back to NY & have Xmas with Joe! Oh, it was so plain. Especially me walking up Taylor Rd from the street car & then when I was in the kitchen.*

Peg was so far away from home and communications were very erratic. Letters came by ship and could take weeks between writing and receiving. She was unaware her family had left Cleveland Heights. The Depression struggles touched the Morrisons, as they did millions of others. The heartbreak of leaving their much-loved house at 1638 Taylor Road was a pain they tried to spare Peg, since she was so far away. Unbeknown to her, the family had already moved into an apartment on Dellenbaugh Avenue in Cleveland. She did not learn about the move until shortly before the new year.

Christmas Eve

Just a short note to tell you Marguerite and I have just celebrated Xmas Eve alone at home. We have a precious tree and we had coffee, sandwiches, Danish cookies, fruit & stuffed dates. We have 3 red candles burning on our table and the candles on the tree. Of course, they are all burned down now, but the big red ones I'm writing by—they're still going. Marguerite & I were the only sober ones in the theatre today & by Finale tonight we were the only 2 who could stand solidly on our feet. We didn't have a drop even though we were offered bottles! I just can't down the stuff. That's all!

Before the year ended, Peg's apprehensions about Mistinguett were confirmed. "It still gives me the willies," Peg exclaimed as she recounted. "She summoned me to her dressing room and that's where she offered me stardom. She said she'd made Maurice Chevalier and Fernandahl both stars and she could make me a star. She invited me to come live at her home and I'd have the use of her limousine, etc. I don't remember exactly how I responded, but the next day I planned my return to the States. Arranged for my passage on the ship and all that."

Friday, Dec. 29

By the time you get this letter I will have sailed. Let's see, this goes the 3rd on the Ile de France & arrives in NY the 10th & you'll get it the 11th. I sail January 10th on the SS Champlain and arrive Jan. 17.

Please don't tell anyone the real reason why I'm coming home. Just say I couldn't stand it another week over here and that I was not earning hardly enough to live on.

This is the real reason, but don't even tell the family. I've got to leave the Folies—or else! If you get what I mean. They like me too well & probably in a year or 2 I could be a big principal [star] thru Mistinguett & the big directors, but I would rather leave. They've been at me and at me, every blasted one of them and finally told me if I didn't care to cooperate I could leave. I can't put up with that Mom. I'd rather go back to NY and do 4 shows a day at Paramount. Mistinguett has been marvelous to me & all that, but she evidently wants to be paid for it. God all mighty, Mom, I'm a nervous wreck. I'll be SO GLAD to leave & get back where men & women are ladies & gentlemen!

I wish I could call you up but I don't know your phone or if you'll have one. I only hope you're all well by now—and for heavens sakes don't worry about me. There's nothing to worry about.

All my love & I'll see you as soon as I can.

A SHOW BIZ MARRIAGE
1934

Sadly, only one letter survived from this year, and Peg's memories of this particular time blurred through the years. She returned to the United States, and to Joe Ancona, arriving in New York City on January 17. Joe was the sax-playing beau she'd left behind when she sailed for Europe thirteen months earlier. Two months later, on March 17, she married Joe Ancona in New York City. The ceremony was performed by Dr. Meldrom who had previously been at the Old Stone Presbyterian Church in Cleveland, Peg's home church. The night before the wedding, Peg wired her sister, Ruth.

> *"Can't come home this weekend but will call tomorrow night at 9 or 10 have everyone there. You answer phone first and don't worry. My love to everyone. Will get home as soon as I can. Peggy"*

She kept her promise and phoned home to tell her family she'd married Joe.

Family had always been important to Peg, and having been so far away for over a year, she was anxious to help wherever she could.

***

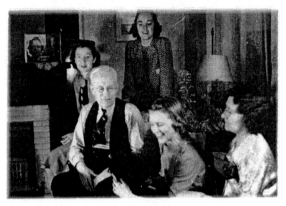

Morrison clan
l to r Betty, Tom, Mary, Peg & Florence

***

Over sixty years later her sisters Betty and Mary provided some vivid memories of 1934.

Betty, who had recently completed cosmetology school, came to New York for an extended stay that spring. She worked in a salon on Washington Square and lived with Peg and Joe in their apartment near the Hudson River. "I was thrilled to be in New York with Peg and Joe," she recalled. "His hours were different from hers and sometimes I'd meet her after a show. I remember going with them to his family's home for dinner on Henry Street." Betty stayed until early summer.

Their baby sister, Mary, prepared for high school graduation in Pompano, Florida. She had spent that school year with her Robinson relatives. Mary remembered, "I had a very difficult time with the move from Taylor Road. The move was difficult on everyone. The Robinsons offered to help by having me come down there."

After graduation, in June 1934, Mary returned to Cleveland and went to work with her sister, Ruth, at the bus company. Betty recalled that she returned home then to care for her father while the others worked.

Their eldest sister, Ruth, is now deceased, so her recollections are not included here. Mary recalled what an important figure Ruth was in her life. "Ruth was like a second mother to me. She helped me with homework, made sure I washed behind my ears, and incessantly corrected our grammar...Betty's and mine. She gave Betty and me $1 each week for lunch money. She was very necessary to me."

In an October letter Peg wrote to Betty about an unusual audition.

> *Well tonight was the night. I wore my red formal and get there to find out you must make a short speech to the audience. So, I had mine all made up. "Good evening ladies & gentlemen. All I wish to say is that I'm really not superstitious but I'm going to keep my fingers crossed anyway—until this is over-- Thank you." Oh I had it down pat—and the last moment when the man brought each girl on stage he asked her name, address, occupation & why we would like to go to Hollywood. Of course I have a corker of an address & I can't say that street name!* [Dellenbaugh Ave.] *More fun! Then I said I was a dancer. He asked if I was working & I said I was until "Saluta" closed. (I got a hand.) Then as to why I wanted to go to Hollywood, I said I'd like to go so I could see the Rocky Mts on the way & that got a big laugh. I wasn't asked for the 2nd round of questions backstage so I don't have a thought of being chosen.*

"Saluta," starring Milton Berle, ran for only two weeks on Broadway.

Peg worked more regularly than Joe did that year.

Nothing very memorable, a variety of steady line ups and some modeling. She sent money home when she could manage it, tried to build some savings and pay for the furniture they needed. As a musician, Joe's work was more erratic than Peg's. Show business now had to support the two of them.

Perhaps the letters disappeared and the memories have faded because it was a difficult year. Marriage to Joe had been a mistake. One that would haunt Peg for several years to come.

BACK ON THE ROAD
1935

Peg and Joe tried to settle into a normal married life. Their careers in show business presented a real challenge. They had a small apartment in Brooklyn where Peg cooked meals, attended baby showers, and carried out the traditional activities of a young wife in the '30s. They worried about paying their bills, and tried to scrape together enough money for a vacation. But the lure of the stage was a powerful force. In a letter to her sister, Ruth, she writes:

> *Wednesday, June 12*
>
> *Oh I have the wanderlust so badly now. I saw the kids off to South America yest'y. You know Danny sent 8 girls down to Rio to the Hotel Copacabana—$40 a wk in Amer. currency & contract for 6 wks—option for 7. It takes them 13 days to get there. Gee I almost cried when Iris broke down saying goodbye to me. It's the loveliest boat—SS Pan American—and they have private baths even in tourist class. Oh it was so thrilling. Three of our kids went. We sent them a big bon voyage basket. They sailed at noon yest'y. I was so jealous. I could have gone—he was begging for blonds. But, of course, I wouldn't dare even mention it or consider it. You know me though, when it comes to travel and adventure. I'm sure I must have some gypsy in me somewhere. Everybody is going places...it's no wonder I've got the itch!*

I guess this show is a 2 weeker, the next picture is Joan Crawford in "No More Ladies" and that's 2 wks for sure and maybe 3.

Later that month she reported to her mother, *"Joe's not working at all now."*

Peg poured her heart out in a letter, written between shows, and mailed to her mom at work.

Saturday, June 29

It's been hotter than Hades the past week and almost unbearable. Perfectly awful for toe work too. My old dead dogs "ain't what they used to was," I guess. This weather makes each foot feel like one huge boil.

Mom, I'm sending this to the library so you don't have to show it to the family. I'm just going to pour out everything to you and I hope you will answer this and send the answer to the Capitol Theater. Don't mention any "troubles" in any letter sent to Joe & me or even to me alone, at the apt., because of course he reads them all.

Well, I'll begin at the beginning. When I first met Joe & went with him those 5 months before going to Paris, I was so much in love with him he absolutely had NO faults in my eyes. Then I went away and the same Joe— errorless—stayed in my mind when I was gone. I came back & we just went together 3 months [actually, it was only two] *and then got married. Pretty soon I began to see his short-comings, but gave him the benefit of the doubt. But now I am absolutely at my wits end.*

Before we were married he told me several little white lies, 2 trivial, one important, now. First he told me he was born here, which doesn't really make much difference, he's naturalized now. Then he told me a long story about a job he had as musician on a boat that went to Berlin or somewhere in Germany, and that he flew from Berlin to Hamburg—some fairy tale—which was nothing important but still, a lie. The important thing is, he told me he graduated from high school. And there's the rub. He never went to high school, and he certainly speaks like it. How he'll ever get on in the business world is beyond me. He uses such poor English that he really embarrasses me when we're with anyone. Not only that, but he can't talk or transact anything—he gets nervous & stutters & can't get anything out. The other night we went to the Paramount, and after he bought the tickets the barker said something about only 35 minutes left of the last feature, so we wanted to get our money back. We had to go in and see the ass't mgr. & do you think Joe could ask—oh no, he hands me the tickets & I was furious. So I had to do all the talking while he stood there like a numbskull!

One trouble with me is that I just can't fight or argue or start a discussion like—about anything like that, because he always takes it wrong, and I can't stand arguments. Mother, this is what scares me—Joe will never be able to support me. I know now. What to do about it is beyond me. If he ever did connect with the Insurance job or Sears Roebuck—the only 2 places he has connections, how could he sell insurance, when he can't even speak to me, without getting nervous and stammering, when I do absolutely nothing to make him nervous. I've never even mentioned it to him, or showed any signs of noticing it.

Well, that's the beginning of my story, but it's not all. He's been out of work for about 3 weeks now. He's had a card to take over to Sears R. in Bklyn & he still hasn't gone. He just helps spend and plan my salary every wk. I pay rent—I pay all, *and gosh darn it I'm thru. I've bot [sic] the furniture, & paid for all we've done or had and what he's earned wouldn't even amount to what we've spent just to* live, *not counting rent or bills. That's just why I got my permanent. He didn't like it very much, that I decided to get one cause it meant $8 + $1 tip. But I got it* anyhow! *A couple of weeks ago when we were pretty strapped he played a horse—a sure fire—and the horse dragged in on the tail end. He didn't tell me he played it till later on—about 1 wk after.*

He used to be pretty good about cleaning house, but the place lately has gone to rack & ruin. The bathroom I insist on having clean. Ashes are all over, pools behind the sink, wet *towels in the hamper, rolls of dust around on the floor, everything filthy. For 2 days last wk I tried to get him to clean it. Finally Sun night I got home & saw it still untouched. I flew off the handle. Oh, he'd gone to the ball game—he couldn't clean. Of course, I should do it I suppose. I do every g-d thing. I bring home the bacon and transact all the business. I suppose it's only right for him to sit on his can and let me do all the cleaning too. It's really funny how I never realized any of these things. Love certainly is blind, that's the truest of any saying!*

I began realizing all this about last summer, but not really seriously until about 6 wks ago. Now, this past wk I've been a wreck. I can't even stand to have him near *me. And another thing is that his demands of me as a wife are entirely too much. I can't stand it—and he's making it so I'll soon hate him.*

Mom, please forgive me for pouring all this out to you, but I don't know who to talk to. I'm just frantic & I simply refuse to go on much longer like this. Maybe I could stand it if at least there were a future for us, but there isn't, there never will be. And by golly, I can do a lot more with my $35 a wk and do a lot better by it than supporting a man and giving all the luxuries of life to him. I could give a few luxuries to myself for a change—get a decent bank account.

I hope you'll answer this as soon as possible, and don't fret over the situation too much. There's no need for you to worry about it. I'd just like you to either advise me or else look for some light on the subject. And for heavens sake don't mention anything at all pertaining to trouble in any of the letters sent to the apt. Write me at the theater— 50th St. & B'way.

Oh, something else I just tho't of. You know Jack, his brother in law. One day last summer we dropped Joe off for work & Jack was driving me home. We were discussing Joe and somehow or other Jack came out with this "Joe says you had money when you were married." It surprised me at the time but didn't sink in. Now I see thru that. Yes, I had a bank account—that was just hunky-dorry—then we ate that up. Then we ate up that paid up insurance policy gift of yours. Then we ate up every bank account I've had since. And we're eating the present one up every lay-off I have. It's gone down just $125 from what it was. So that's that Mom. What do you make out of it?

Peg mailed that letter on Sunday. The following day she wired her mother at the library, *"Don't worry all discussed last night everything understood letter follows."* This crisis passed, but the Ancona marriage was on a rocky road.. The only thing that changed was the size of the rocks.

> *Monday, July 8*
>
> *It's so hot here it's unbearable & doing 3 dances a show, I feel as if I'm back in non-stop variety in London— and we wear everything but the kitchen sink and I don't know how they messed up on that! And the toe shoes— heavens—instead of standing straight up on them, we're on about a 45° angle—on account of the heat!*

Early in August, Joe and Peg gave up their apartment in Brooklyn and went to Cleveland for a little R&R. When they returned to New York, they moved in with Joe's family. By the end of August, Peg was in rehearsal for an American Folies Bergère, which went on tour, opening in Boston on August. 29th.

> *Wed, Aug. 21 Brooklyn*
>
> *Well, I can't wait until this one more wk is over and we get on our way. I'll be so glad to get a little money in my fist that I don't have to shell out here and there. I should buy a different trunk, mine is so full of moths that I'm afraid to put anything in it, and I can't even afford a mere $10 or $15, whatever it'd be 2nd hand. My bank account is down to just enough for me to take to Boston until we get pd. And I'm the only one worrying. It's more fun!*

The American Folies opened at the RKO Boston Theater to rave reviews. Peg's first letter home was full of enthusiasm.

Sunday, Sept. 1

Thank heavens all the ordeal of opening is over now and everything is going quite nicely. The managers are all beaming, and why shouldn't they—sensational newspaper comments & people standing at all performances. They took in $6000 the opening day, $7500 yest'y and it'll be more today because there're 5 shows today. The people applaud, shout and enjoy it more thoroughly than I've ever seen any audience devour anything. I'm getting along swell in the show. It's really the best break I ever had because I really do something like in the Chopin Ballet. I just love it.

Later that week she reported that the theater had broken all records that week, grossing $38,000.

The American Folies Bergère closed in Indianapolis on Dec 13, 1935, after a 15-week run that took them to Providence, Rhode Island; Columbus, Ohio; Cleveland, Chicago, Minneapolis, Davenport and Cedar Rapids, Iowa; Kansas City, Detroit and Youngstown, Ohio. The Morrison clan continued their tradition to catch her shows when Peg was nearby. Her sisters, Mary and Ruth, made it up to Detroit, and her mom and sister Betty joined a number of friends from Cleveland who motored down to Youngstown.

Wednesday, Dec. 4 Youngstown

Say, [Betty] you are the talk of the 3 of us, Te, Tea & me. Those date nut bars are the most delicious things I ever ate or they ever ate. Really, honey they are delicious. We dived into them tonight & made it our night lunch with a container of coca cola each.

Throughout the road trip, Peg's marriage to Joe Ancona

continued to unravel. When the Folies ended, she asked her mom to tell the rest of the family that she wouldn't join Joe in Philadelphia.

In September, when the show played Columbus, Peg and her roommate, Chula, went together and bought a black Scottie puppy. Bobo became the delight of her life. He entertained the troupe with his antics, slept in a box in her berth on the Pullman, and gave her that unconditional love so helpful in easing the pain of a disintegrating marriage. When Chula left the troupe in November, Peg paid Chula her share of the dog, $12.50. Now she had Bobo all to herself!

On December 14, 1935, Peg and Bobo returned to New York City and took up residence in the Knickerbocker Hotel. It quickly became apparent that she would have to look for more economical accommodations, so Peg decided to rent a room in the Bronx from the Muller's, the family of her roommate, Marguerite, from Paris days. The only down side was that she had to send Bobo home to Cleveland.

By year's end, Joe was working hard to woo her back. He wired that he was coming to spend New Year's Eve with her. And, Peg "thought" she was in rehearsal for a job opening the first week in January at the Paramount in Newark, New Jersey. Her plan was to commute to Newark from the Muller's place in the Bronx. However, she'd heard an ugly rumor that the job was a phony—that something else was opening at the Paramount the next week.

Rumors proved true. The Paramount job did not pan out. Peg faced a new year filled with uncertainty. What would 1936 bring?

CAPTIVATING RIO
1936

Peg agreed to give the marriage another try and returned to Philadelphia with Joe right after the new year began. She refused, however, to tolerate his deceit, and by mid-January, was back in New York, living at the Muller's home and looking for work.

Good fortune smiled on Peg again. She answered a call for auditions and was asked to rehearse for a new show being assembled by Earl Leslie. Following several days of rehearsals selections would be made, and she hoped to be among the girls who were chosen. Peg was excited about the prospects of a new show, but enjoyed piquing her family's curiosity by not revealing too much about it.

Saturday, Jan. 25 New York

It is such a temptation to tell you what I'm rehearsing for but I guess I'll just have to restrain the desire until Mon. But I'll give you another hint & probably from that, you'll know. If, I get it, I will sail *3 weeks from today and be on the water 19 days. Now, don't tell* anyone. *I'm hoping I get it—and I think I've a pretty good chance, but of course, one never* knows until it's all signed. If *I* don't get it, well, I'm not supposed to get it, and I won't feel badly. But naturally it'll be a perfectly marvelous experience if it happens.*

I have to laugh at all the "ifs" in this letter. Another

if—If I get it, will you by hook or by crook come to NY to see me off?

Well, now that you practically know where the job is for—I'll let you guess for a day or 2 and I'll write you Monday and tell you yes or no. I can just see you looking up to see how long it takes to get from NY to anywhere.

Pleasant dreams and just remember that what will be, will be. I do all in my power, but the rest is in someone else's hands.

Monday brought good news.

Monday, Jan. 27

At last I can tell you what "it's" about. The picking was today and I was the 1st one picked after the captain. As usual, don't *tell anyone outside the family until I say because we have to get our passports before we sign contracts. I'm going down tomorrow to get mine renewed.*

It's for Buenos Aires, S. America and we work in a theater there for 3 months and then go to a Casino in Rio for 4 to 6 weeks after. In Sept, he [Mr. Leslie] *has the Casino de Paris in Paris, France and would like to keep this show together for Paris but of course, that's not definite, so I don't count on it.*

We have to pay for our own passports and tips on the boat, but I don't care—it's seeing some more of the world.

It's a very *reliable office that's sending the show. The office must have a bond in a bank here before they can take girls out of the country.*

We sail on the S/S Western World, Munson Line, Sat, Feb. 15 and arrive in B.A. March 4. I'll let you know as soon as we sign contracts and then *you can tell anyone you want.*

A couple of days later, Peg shares with her sister, Betty, the red tape involved.

> *Yesterday I got my passport renewed and today I had to go to Police Headquarters and get a certificate that I've never been in jail. They take fingerprints of each finger and look up to see if you have a "record" and then when they find you have none, they give you this certificate all signed with the City seal and the rt. thumb fingerprint of the party in question and you leave—one errand finished.*
>
> *Then I had to go to a doctor and get a certificate that he had examined me—that I had been vaccinated—had no infections or venereal diseases and that I was in normal health. Then I had to take that certificate down to the City Dept. of Health and get it OK'd and signed and "sealed" by the City.*
>
> *That ends my running around, so I expect to sign my contact tomorrow. I'll let you know as soon as I do.*

Saturday, February 15, 1936, the SS Western World set sail from New York, bound for Buenos Aires with stops at Bermuda, Rio de Janiero, Santos and Montevideo. On board was Earl Leslie's new show, including Peggy Morrison, headed for Teatro Casino in Buenos Aires. None of the Morrison clan made it to New York to see her off this time. Money was too tight.

The long voyage provided Peg the opportunity to seal new friendships, among them, one with the ship's Radio Officer,

Charlie Stewart. Though Charlie was smitten with the leggy dancer from Cleveland, she was technically a married woman and insisted their friendship be just that. "We remained friends, just friends, for several years. I saw Charlie frequently over the years as he was in and out of New York, for as long as I was in show business," Peg reflected.

The voyage also meant many new experiences, all of which were recorded in a lengthy diary.

> Last night was the first night we could see the "Southern Cross" among the stars. It's really lovely. After the movie, Sunny [a fellow dancer who would become Peg's roommate] and I pulled our deck chairs away back on deck and just sat and looked at the stars—what an array! Honestly, it's so different from the summer sky of USA—the "Milky Way" really looks like a stream of milk—and the stars dot the ENTIRE sky way down to the horizon. I mean it! We crossed the Equator this past Monday at 4:23 AM. Earlier today I caught sight of land…Brazil, I'm told. There was the most picturesque sail boat with 3 big white sails between our ship and land. The sky was blue, the water bluer, the ocean as smooth as glass, the sun shining in full glory and oh! What a thrill.

Following the Rio stopover:

> I have so much to tell you about Rio that I doubt if I ever could put it down or even try to express it. The sight was so gorgeous that all I wanted to do was to sit and think and just look. There are mountains of all sizes and shapes, water in every scene, palm trees, and everything that makes pictures what they are! Sunny's friends met us at the boat and showed us around.

They drove us up to Jaoa, and Mom, you never saw anything like it. The road up there was a perfect thrill in itself, but the biggest thrill was when we got there to just look out over the view and relax. On the way up we passed beautiful trees with clusters of purple flowers and other trees with pink flowers that had half fallen to the road. Waaaay below is the ocean.

They do have some strange food in Brazil. One is quite a delicacy made from the inside of palm trees. It's called "palmetta"...tastes something like asparagus.

I think I've never spent such an enjoyable day. I would most certainly like to live there!

The next day we stopped in Santos...what a contrast! Santos is such an old town and so quaint and dirty and Rio is so modern. Santos reminded me of a little old French town.

Wednesday, March 4

Just a PS to tell you that we are in BA now and are safely located in a pension which is all arranged for us. It was done by the girl who was in Paris with me and who married a very wealthy man here. Buenos Aires is very nice. I like it much better than I thought I would. The theater is simply the last word in loveliness. Is it MODERN and practically new. It's like Fall here now. We start rehearsing at 8 tonight and probably will keep on until we open Friday night. We will do three shows at the theatre starting at 7 PM , then 9 and 11. Then we do one show (one number) at the Club about 1—and we are through.

To her family back in Ohio, there was something more ominous about Peg's being in South America than there had been when she was in Europe. Stories of danger to foreigners peppered the news at home. In a letter written a few days after their arrival, responding to an air mail letter from home, she endeavored to put their minds at ease.

> *Now first of all about your little worry about me here. It used to be very dangerous here. But now, all that "traffic" has been cleared out and foreigners from the States have* Police protection *now—which they didn't used to have. It isn't any more dangerous than NY. So don't worry. Friends of Sunny's have told friends of theirs here to look her up, so we also have good American friends here who escort us anywhere we want to go. We haven't bought a meal yet! They made a general clean-up on the city within the past 6 months & are very particular about everything.*

> *We moved from the pension and are now living at a hotel very near the theatre where the rest of the company is staying.*

> *Yesterday we started rehearsing at 2 PM, had time off for dinner, then rehearsed right thru the night (in costumes) & got home at 7 AM! I've just gotten up, but wanted to get this in tomorrow's departure.*

Peg exhibited some subtle signs of maturity during her time in South America. First, she committed to sending letters to her family twice a week. Airmail often took two weeks or more to reach Cleveland. She was also faithful about sending letters regularly via boat mail. However, her letters increasingly addressed cares and concerns for her stateside family, rather than accounts of her own experiences...except to share her excitement.

Sunday, March 22 [her 25th birthday]

*I have so much to tell you I hope I can get it on paper!
I didn't say anything about my birthday to the kids, but
when the cable came from René,* [Calderon, a friend from
Paris] *Sunny wrote down the date, etc. Well, last night
the last finale of the last show when everyone was on stage,
(it was after midnight) they had it planned, and on a
certain step everyone hollered together, "Happy Birthday,
Peggy!" WELL!!! I could hardly finish the dance; it went
right to my legs. They all said afterward that they were so
excited about it waiting for that step to come, that they were
making mistakes. And I have NEVER been so thrilled.
That certainly meant more to me than anything—more
than a priceless gift!*

*When I got up today I was ironing in my gown with
my robe over it. Paula called and asked if I'd come up to
their apt for a special breakfast and to come just the way I
was. So, I went up and she and Toy and Cecil and I had
to have champagne for my birthday breakfast. After we
finished Paula said what a shame we hadn't left anything
for Sunny—she felt so badly but she said she'd come down
with me and tell her she had thought of her anyhow!*

*So, we all came down and I opened the door, and
MOM! All 16 girls were in our apt and yelled "Happy
Birthday!" and there was a HUGE cake in the center
of a table full of food. The cake had "Happy Birthday,
Peggy" on it and candles in the most unique candle holder
you ever saw. Besides all that there were gifts to be opened
and cards as well. Every one of the girls came, and some of
them even broke dates to come. After we cut the cake, (how,
I hated to cut into it) we all got up and either said a poem*

or told a joke or did some stunt in the entertainment line and we sang songs. Oh, it was more fun and certainly a huge success.

Sunny told me afterwards that the kids were so excited about it that they could hardly wait for the day to come. I can't think when I've had such a happy birthday and believe me, it meant so much to me that the girls think that much of me. I know you were all thinking of my birthday and I wish you all could have been at my party and heard the girls holler "Happy Birthday" to me last night.

Now, I want to send a special extra Happy Birthday home to Ruth and Daddy. So, many happy returns to both of you. [Ruth's birthday was April 4, and their father's on April 7.]

Talk of the show's future beyond Buenos Aires spawned an idea for Peg. She revealed it to her parents in a letter dated

Thursday, March 26

I'm going to wait till I get $500 together (which will be about 6 months from now) and you and Daddy will come to Paris on your 2nd honeymoon—and you'll come together if I have to make a court rule you to come! I'm sure the girls would be thrilled for you both and wouldn't mind being left alone for a couple of months. They have their lives to live yet and someday I'll do the same for them. This time though, if I get to Paris and if things turn out as I see them, you and Daddy must make the trip. I swear I'm so thrilled thinking about it, I can't sleep. The $500 will cover return passage for you both, passports, tips and leave plenty for new clothes. What do you say, is it a go? You'd better say yes.

Gee all I can think of is you and Daddy on the boat, coming to Paris. Sunny & I will have an apt. ready and oh we'll have a marvelous time. Now, Mother & Daddy, I don't want to hear you say, "oh no, the money can be used to pay off the mortgage" or some such thing. When I'm in Paris (if I get there of course), is the time for you to have the trip and I don't want any back talk from either of you. My sole aim now is working for the family, and first of all to give you and Daddy a vacation like you've never had in your life. So, get busy and do a little imagining.

A letter to her sister, Ruth, described challenges for young women in Argentina.

Monday, April 6

The sidewalks are so narrow that 2 people only can walk comfortably, but you have to split up to pass anyone. And talk about "gooses" in Paris—well, they're nothing compared to good old Argentina "gooses." Boy they get you coming and going. If you are walking along & 2 men are walking towards you, they split & pass one on each side of you. One gets a good feel of your crotch and the other of your lungs! Some fun for them! One day I got fed up and hauled off & socked a fellow who gave me a "rub down" when Sunny & I were looking in a shop window. Well, the fellow was so dumbfounded he turned around & his mouth just fell open!

As their time at Teatro Casino wound down the troupe wrestled with the uncertainty of "where next." Talk of doing a couple weeks in Rio, then Johannesburg, South Africa and then on to Marseille and Paris, alternated with rumors that they would return directly to NY. The uncertainty persisted to the very end.

Sunday, June 7 (rec'd June 16)

When you read this, I'll be on a boat going somewhere, but I couldn't tell you where it'll be. Isn't that awful? It's probably some shock to you. I'll tell you what. If we hear we are going to work in Rio or France, I'll cable you, so in that case you would already have rec'd a cable by the time you read this. If we come to NY I'll be able to see Ruth & Mary off to Bermuda 3 days after I get back! Do you think Bobo will know me??

Peg's prediction was true. They sailed from Buenos Aires on Saturday, June 13, just three-and-a-half months after they had arrived. In spite of all the rumors and stories, the post Buenos Aires bookings had not materialized. The troupe was headed home to New York.

Sunday, June 14 Aboard S/S American Legion—at sea

We had the most perfect send off! Our farewell started the night before. We 3, [Peg, Sunny & their friend Jeanne] went out formal, did the round of all the clubs and got "just gay" enough. We danced and danced. First time in a coon's age for me and everyone in the party made it known in each place we went that I was the crack dancer. Everyone danced again & again with me & it kind of embarrassed me for the other kids, but I sure had one swell time.

Saturday, Jeanne's friend took us to the boat. All our friends were there and when we saw them all grouped down on the pier it was too much for every one of us. We cried & cried. I tho't my heart would break. Then I saw the good old Stars & Stripes waving and that finished me. I SOBBED. Even the little "clappers" [boys who were hired by the theatre to applaud] *were down to say goodbye—the dressers—everyone. Everything had been so perfect, the send off, the parting celebration the night before and everything.*

Soon after they arrived in Argentina, Jeanne met a wealthy man who "took a shine" to her. According to Peg, "He made an arrangement with her that he'd never, ever touch her, but he wanted to be her friend, buy her gifts, do nice things for her. Whenever he took her out, Sunny & I were to go along to make sure he wasn't taking advantage of Jeanne. So we did. The three of us were living 'high on the hog.' We had a grand time, thanks to Jeanne's friend."

Wednesday, June 17 Santos, Brazil

We docked in Santos yesterday AM. It was a beautiful sight. Mts, islands, more mts, and it took us quite a time to get up the river, or bay, or whatever it is, and into the pier. After lunch we set out for Sao Paulo. Made a dicker with the cab driver for $14 round trip. After about 2 miles we started climbing the mts. Boy, that old rickety cab went up that mt. in 2nd and we couldn't hear each other talk. We climbed higher and higher—passing trucks—going just fine—around a hairpin curve and I mean a hairpin curve every 50 or 75 ft. it seemed. We finally got to the top (3200 ft) and stopped to let the engine cool. You NEVER saw such a sight. Miles down was Santos, the ocean, little rivers, it looked like we were in a plane.

Thursday, June 25

This is Mary's birthday & I'm going to try and send a radiogram if it isn't too expensive.

Late last night we took the victrola up on the sun deck. We lay down on deck chair cushions, played gorgeous music and watched the stars. Talk about shooting stars! It looked like the heavens were celebrating the 4th of July. And on every one I wished I'd go back to Rio very soon. I wished it so many times it's bound to come true!

Day before yesterday we passed the mouth of the Amazon River. Of course, we couldn't see it but the ocean was such a terrible color—very muddy, etc & they say it's from the Amazon feeding into the ocean.

A day-stop at the island of Trinidad and a visit to an Anglican School gave Peg yet another look at life outside the United States.

As we entered, all the children stood up and we were met by the assistant principal who was to show us through the school. It consisted of one large room with all classes together, each one having their own section. The children were seated along benches so close together that it was remarkable how they kept such good discipline. We were shown the children's handy work such as woven baskets and trays and pieces of embroidery work, and also their composition and arithmetic notebooks. We were very impressed by our warm welcome and the manner in which education is carried on. There wasn't a white person in this Anglican school.

The S/S American Legion docked in New York on July 1, 1936. Another overseas odyssey completed.

With five years experience under her belt, Peg was optimistic about the forthcoming job hunt.

Wednesday, July 8 New York

Yesterday I bo't [sic] a lovely new dress and it did the trick. I landed a job in it today! For Boots McKenna— Montreal. Remember, he did the dances for "Saluta?" Well, he thinks I'm the last word.

As so often happened, it didn't materialize.

Sunday, July 19

Well, I had a lovely letter all written but I tore it up because I immediately found out it was worthless. It was all about Montreal, etc—and now I'm not going to Montreal. Guess the boss from the Chez—who did the picking—didn't think I was a "club" type. Sunny is going but she hates to go without me. I told her not to be silly—she needs the job and she should take it. I don't feel the least bit badly about not getting picked though, because I evidently wasn't supposed to go. So, I feel perfectly sure I'll find something even better.

Saturday, July 25

Oh how I wish I might come home and be with you on your vacation! But I must keep doing the "rounds" and get myself a job. There are plenty of shows being cast now but just try *to get in! You have to be a personal friend of President Roosevelt almost!*

I had one terrible disappointment this last wk. But,

I didn't even cry—that's how well I stood it. I know now that everything happens for the best and my job will come soon. The disappointment was a job for the Folies Bergère in Paris. There are 8 girls going—sailing a wk from today, and they are short one girl. I had an interview with Josephine Baker's mgr. last Tues. and he said I'd be fine except they want a redhead. I told him I could easily become one. He seemed very pleased with me and said he'd call, but no call, so that's that.

Don't worry about me. I'm happy and in the peak of health & I'll land a job soon. You see if I don't!

And, by mid-August she did have the job.

Tuesday, Aug 18

We are rehearsing very hard and long now but I LOVE it. Costume fittings besides. Company rehearsals every night and group rehearsals afternoons—fittings in the morning.

Variety says we don't open until Sept 1st because the place isn't completed yet. I believe it too. The show could be ready but there'd have to be plenty of rehearsing to open by next Wed.

A few days later...

Saturday, Aug. 22

The biggest and saddest news is that our opening is postponed until Sept. 8. That's 2 wks from next Wed. So there's nothing for us to do but to wait. We don't get any salary until we start to work. We can draw, but of course it's taken out gradually from our salaries. But, I'm not worried. Reason for postponement—the stage fell in! They built an ordinary stage and then put 15 tons of revolving stage on it and now it all has to be rebuilt!

Joe's coming in tomorrow to see me. I think we can talk the whole thing over sensibly and come to some understanding. At any rate, I have nothing against him, and no hatred or anything like that in my heart. I know Joe pretty well I think, and I believe he'll listen to reason, a plan I have and am going to present to him. This is it.

I'll be in NY 6 months. If I could use the furniture for as long as I'll be in NY, I would then give it to him to do with as he wished. Then I would have some use out of it and could enjoy it myself—have a place of my own for $35 a month—and save.

As 1936 drew to a close, Peg was working at Shea's Hippodrome Theater in Toronto, Canada. She remembered winning a bingo jackpot there and using the proceeds to make her first plane trip...back to New York for a visit.

OPENING NEW YORK'S INTERNATIONAL
CASINO
1937

The Toronto job at Shea's Hippodrome Theater continued through the early part of the year.

Thursday aft., April 1 Toronto

Last night in the flower parade I got so much applause—my goodness! They all must have been drunk! Every time we went around when I got to the front there was a big outburst. I'm a daisy and my costume is black chiffon—a scanty brassiere, a very scanty G-string and a diagonal piece about 1 inch wide of chiffon going from the left of the brassiere to the right of the G-string, and all of it covered with daisies. Then I have a long black chiffon train with daisies and stars on it and I wear a black straw-ish hat—very becoming—wide brim and it has daisies on it. Everyone says I have the prettiest costume. I think so too...

By June, Peg was back in New York, rooming with Sunny, and picking up jobs when she could, doing a few shows and quite a bit of modeling, while she waited for something "good" that would last awhile.

Wednesday, June 2 NYC

Going to a call right now. It's for a steady line up [chorus line] *in Brooklyn. At any rate I work tomorrow & Friday with Sunny.*

Later...Went to call—nothing happened but anyhow I start at B'way Theater with Sunny tomorrow. New show goes in Sat. I jump in this one for 2 days and continue with the new show. At least it'll be a couple of weeks work. Thank heavens.

Friday night, July 2

Well, the theater job we had that was supposed to open on Sunday is postponed until a week from today. So, I am going to see about a job in Hershey, PA for the summer—steady line—work Thurs, Fri & Sat and $20 for the 3 days (4 shows—one on Thurs & Fri and 2 on Sat!!!) They say it's just gorgeous there. Anyhow, I'm sick and tired of hanging on here and waiting for the Apollo Theater to open.

I posed for an artist last night and made $2. It's hard work for one who enjoys jumping around.

We rehearsed for the Apollo Theater yesterday & today & we're so sore and stiff—we kicked until unconscious! They've only been postponing this opening for about 2 weeks! You see they closed all the Burlesque houses and now different people have gotten permits to open those houses and produce Variety shows—something NY doesn't have. It's 2 shows a day, I believe—maybe 3—but it's like the old time vaudeville. Salary is $25 a week. They had such a hard time getting permits that's why all the delay. And of course it isn't burlesque or anything like it but we still feel funny about doing it so all our gang gave phony names! Leaving the place, we back out!

Monday, July 5

I have decided not to go to Hershey. Of course, I haven't heard from the man yet, but I've decided to stay here & take the Apollo and be here *if Germany actually materializes or if Chester Hale has another call or something similar.*

There was an article in the News saying the NY Rockettes were so WONDERFUL in Paris in this 1937 run at the Palais, there was a very serious stampede after them by thousands of people who had watched. They (the people) were so taken with them they all rushed after them & police & military guards just joined in the push and didn't even attempt to keep order! They did only 1 performance (4 numbers) on July 2.

I do hope you all had a glorious weekend. Guess Ruth [who was now working in Indianapolis] *was home—gee how I'd love to be there too.*

Sunday, July 11

I guess the Apollo is really going to open as everyone could draw money last Friday. I wasn't there but I went in yesterday and we were excused until Monday at 2. Everyone can draw again tomorrow so I'll be there and I'll draw. Then we open Friday next. Just as soon as we open then I can draw $10 and I'll send it to you. But now we can only draw $2 at a time.

The Apollo was a good "stop gap," but wasn't what Peg really wanted. She longed to work again for the producers who had taken her to Paris and Buenos Aires.

Finally, there was a call for auditions for an elegant,

swanky, new nightclub opening in New York City. The producer, Jacque Charles, had been at the Paramount in Paris in '32 when Peg was there. "The International Casino, on Broadway, was a very ritzy, dinner/night club featuring a troupe of ballet dancers, a troupe of acrobats, partially nude show girls, stairways emerging from the ceiling," Peg recalled. "It was very elaborate."

Monday night, July 12

Today I went up to see Jacque Charles again.. I had my hair set at 9 AM, went home, had a bath & put fresh, clean, crisp clothes on, and then left to make that good impression. The audition room is like a big ballroom & he and the other men sit way down at the other end from the door. When I came in Jacques Charles saw me & he just beamed from ear to ear. Before I even could say hello to him he said how pretty I was today(!) and my! didn't my hair look lovely!

I told him I had it done especially to have him like it. And he did. Thank heavens. The rehearsals start Wed. at 3 but although I think I have a better than average chance to stay in, it still isn't definite. I imagine Chester Hale will be there Wed. and I sure hope he doesn't have any say in the matter. I don't believe he has, but still, one never knows, does one!

Everything happens at once. The old Burlesque houses have their licenses to reopen as variety shows, (no nudes) and not burlesque, and the one I've been rehearsing for opens for sure on Thurs. night. They rehearse every afternoon. Now I can't rehearse both places at once, nor work all day and make the ballet rehearsals so I went over this afternoon and told Ted I couldn't be in it at least for the first wk. I didn't say why. Then in case I get let out from the International Casino ballet I can go back to the Apollo for the next show next week...

My oh my—I guess they'll never find Amelia Earhart. Andy thinks all those radio messages were fakes except her SOS saying she had only half hr more of gas. Personally, I think she's been devoured by the sharks days ago. But I hope not. She is (or was) a brave woman and a marvelous example of American womanhood.

The Rockettes arrived home today from their great Parisian success. And they started to work tonight again, with much welcoming & celebration, etc.

Peg had been back in the United States for a year, and the issue of her marriage remained unresolved. She and Joe had lived apart for almost two years. Her hope to retrieve the furniture she had purchased and the wedding gifts from her family, drove Peg to try and try again for an amicable split.

Thursday, July 15

Did I tell you I wrote and asked Joe for the furniture & when I didn't receive an answer in 2 or 3 wks, I wrote a card saying "Having always credited you with being a gentleman, I am surprised you don't answer correspondence any more. I'd like an answer by return mail. Peggy."

Yesterday I spent at court from 9-1 trying to get "support." The man was awfully nice to me & said he thought the court couldn't do anything about the furniture, but Joe could be made to support me. I had that call at 3 for International Casino so I waited until 1 and had gone thru only half the red tape necessary and I had to leave. Today I have to go again at 3 for International Casino so I didn't attempt to do the other. However, the first free day I have, I shall spend it at court and all I have to do there is tell THE TRUTH. I would never tell anything else but. And they will make him give me money every week. I figure I'm not asking for anything that doesn't belong to me & I've been so soft so far, he just has me twisted around his little finger. In MY State the home & furniture belongs to the WIFE no matter who paid for it. Whatever court that comes under, I'm going there & I'm going to get MY furniture. Mother, do you think that is wrong to stick up for what is rightfully yours? I've thought and thought about it and I don't feel it is wrong, so long as I don't tell any lies to get anything from him. After all, he is still my husband "officially."

Yesterday the call at 3 PM for Int. Casino was conducted for eliminations. Hale was there just watching! Sandrini, & Bergé & Jacques Charles paid so much attention to me!! There were 9 groups of 8 (that's how many girls were there). I was in the 5th group. He'd take one group at a time and give them a combination. Then each group would get the same combination. Of course, we'd all practice it in back before it came our turn. Well, when group 5 (my group) was called up—all groups stood in a semi-circle and Sandrini & Bergé said "Morrison, stand here"...right in the center of the circle. And Chester Hale right smack in front of me! And we did the combination and boy, I just danced my absolute best. We had about 5 different combinations and some were not so easy.

It was almost time to be excused—we were on the last combination & the 2nd group was doing it. Jacques Charles put on his hat, picked up his cane, walked to the center of the room & beckoned to me. So I went over & he asked if

I was thru yet—what group I was in & I said "5," so he said "oh, you'll be thru in a short time." I said I hoped so because I was going to work and I'd soon have to leave. (I did work last night and made $3.50 modeling.) Well, you think everyone didn't notice that Charles did that? And that I was put in the center front of the group! (and no one in any other group was put there!) Well, I feel I have an excellent chance of staying in but still and all, I am not sure because Moss (financier) has to approve of all girls. At any rate I was told to come back today at 3, and plenty were let go—but quietly and in a way that they weren't embarrassed in front of everyone. So, I'll see what happens today.

Later. . .

Here I am and much *to relate. The combinations today were quite hard. There were 37 there. We only had 3 combinations but spent lots of time on them. Oh, I danced so hard. I went over to get a drink and Charles was sitting there. He said to me, "You are the last one—the shortest one we use. But you are* set.*" Well, I thanked him very much, and went over to sit down. Then they lined up each group and some were told to go to the table—they gave their names & addresses. I was not among them—so I wondered! Then those who were* not *told to go to the table were called together & told to come back tomorrow at 3. So* we *were the ones picked and the others were not.*

The International Casino doesn't open for about one month yet, but as soon as we get set definitely & start rehearsing, *I imagine we'll be able to draw. At any rate, Monday when I see Marguerite I'm going to borrow some more money from her and I'll get enough to send you. That's my only worry. I could have borrowed it before, but I just* hate *to borrow, and I thought maybe I wouldn't have to. Now I will, as long as I have a job in view. Of course, even though Jacques Charles says I'm set, I'll still only believe it when I start working or draw money. But even though he's speaking for me etc, etc, I feel I could stand on my own merits because I know I got all the combinations OK. And I kept myself attractive, and well groomed. But as you see, they are using such tall girls, that I'm the shortest & maybe he is making that much allowance in order to get me in. And I thought I was tall!*

The next day the contract was all signed, sealed and delivered!

Friday night, July16

Even though I wasn't worried, if there had been any worries, they are all over now. Today I signed my contract for the ballet at the International Casino. $40 a week. And it's going to be for 6 months. They selected 14 girls out of very close to 100 that tried out altogether. We don't get paid for rehearsals and it opens in 4 or 5 wks.

I realize I got in thru influence, but, I can do the work and if I couldn't do it I don't think the influence would do any good. This Monsieur Bergé, the ballet master is WONDERFUL. I am in 7th Heaven. I'm so happy! At last, *at long last, I have a job where I can* dance. *And, what beautiful work. It is the loveliest I've ever in my life seen. Real Russian Ballet. My body aches all over, but I love that ache. I have a bruise on the back of my neck from one thing we did a lot yesterday, where we had to throw the head back* very *quickly. So I did it so hard I bruised myself!! I don't care.*

I know you know what a happy heart I have tonight. And I know that Someone takes care of me. I've had to wait for this and get into debt, but it's worth every bit of it. The training I'll get couldn't be bought because he is such an excellent master of the dance. Think of it, 4 or 5 weeks of intensive training and then 6 months work of such gorgeous work. And every day free, all day long—only working at night, 8:30 & 11:30. I am so grateful, so thankful, so happy...

Wouldn't it be wonderful if you could attend the opening night of the International Casino...

Rehearsals for the International Casino began. The euphoria over this incredible opportunity was dampened somewhat by the persisting negotiations with Joe.

Monday night, July 19

Yes, Mom, I already wrote Joe once and offered a compromise. I'd pay the $40 storage due [for the furniture] *if he'd sign it over to me to dispose of it, half to his mother & half to me. He NEVER so much as answered to say "no." It was just plain silence.*

You know as well as I that his sister isn't going to use that furniture, nor are they paying the storage. It's not that I want to doubt Joe's word, but figure it out for yourself. His sister has a house *full of nice furniture. Where they'd ever put it is beyond me. And what they'd ever* want *it for is also out of the question. They have a fireplace in the house (and they "own" and won't be moving). They have plenty of chairs, and they couldn't use that modern furniture* *with their stuff anyhow. He has a girl friend and is only marking time until I cough up $300 and set him free. Then they'll use the furniture that I worked pretty hard to get. It's quite plain.*

However, I'll write him again, a nice letter, and ask him to weigh the whole thing on a scale of right & wrong & see if we can't come to some agreement. Of course, I won't even hint that I'm considering court action. Then he'd never come to NY.

My soreness is all gone, but my insides feel as if they've dropped 3 inches, so tomorrow I'm going to invest in a dance belt. Believe me, I'm squeezing those nickels till the Buffalos yell! Maybe I'll get a couple of modeling jobs like I've had. They sure help.

Rehearsals continued through July and August. The four or five weeks preparation before the opening stretched into 8...10 weeks...all without pay! Meanwhile, negotiations with Joe continued.

Sunday, Aug. 22

Joe arrived at 5:30 AM and I hadn't slept a wink. Just wasn't tired or sleepy. So, we went out to Childs and talked over a cup of tea. It was very easy talking to him. This is the result—I am getting $10 a wk from him until my first salary. (that is what I asked for) and I am getting the furniture to use as long as I'm in NY. So I'll get my apt. Of course, that'll be after I open and get on my feet. And he is going to get the divorce. After I open he'll take me to Phila. for an hour or 2—just long enough for the lawyer or sheriff to present me with divorce procedure papers and then I come back & when I don't appear at the trial to *contest it, he gets the divorce—on grounds of desertion. It's OK with me.*

Before he left, Joe gave me $5 and said he'd mail the other $5 tomorrow. Asked all about the family etc and for Bobo. We had a very nice talk...

Postponements of the opening continued. It was scheduled for September 15...then September 17... Modeling jobs kept the bill collectors at bay.

Sunday night, Sept 12

We don't open tomorrow, or did you guess it? We open next Friday, Sept 17. Will let you know as soon as we find out the next date after that! Personally, we've decided they're saving it for the World's Fair in '39!

I worked for that artist Friday—3 hours, $3—an original of me in my new suit. Oh, was I thrilled with it. Wish I could have it!

Finally, the anticipation reached its climax. A clipping from the *New York Daily Mirror*, Friday, Sept. 17, 1937, related:

"Tonight's the Night...that brings a new standard of dining and after-dark entertainment to Broadway and the world, at the thrilling opening of New York's greatest revue restaurant and adjoining salons. International Casino...44th to 45th Streets on Broadway."

Thursday night—late, Sept. 16

We rehearsed last night from 7 PM straight thru

until 7 this morning. Can you imagine that? I have to be in at 11 AM tomorrow. We'll go right thru the show twice—have 3 hours off for dinner and our OPENING show is at 10 PM. All tonight we worked on the Sun Ballet—my favorite. I could weep just from the thrill of that entire scene. Well, the entire show as far as that goes. I just can't believe we are opening after all these weeks. Will write again tomorrow night after the big opening. Oh boy! At last*! At* long *last!*

It was a bittersweet occasion. The elaborate production depended on a complex set of mechanics...revolving stages... staircases dropping from the rafters...intricate maneuvers on which the dancers relied.

Saturday afternoon, Sept. 18

We opened but only about 1/3 of the show went on. Bergé said we could have put on a show like that Aug 25! Mr. Sandrini & Charles cried. Nothing worked yesterday afternoon. So we had one *production number & all the acts worked in front of the curtain. No time now to go into details. Rehearsal right now. More tears were shed among the company than anyone can imagine. There's somethin' fishy going on. I'd bet any amount that there is one or more in that mechanical "crew" of men that is being paid off by the French Casino to gum up our works. Every "accident" has NOT been accidental but deliberate. And why, when the night before EVERYTHING worked and yesterday aft. NOTHING worked. The place was jammed to capacity. More notables than you can shake a finger at—Clark Gable, Conrad Nagel, Jack Dempsy, Roosevelts—oh it was awful! They expect to give the* complete *show Monday. Until then we work as last night. I do 2 numbers, "Harmony" and "Polka." Am dying to see if the critics were lenient.*

All guests there last night are invited to return within 2 weeks to see the COMPLETE show free of charge. Incidentally, what we did *went over MARVELOUSLY.*

Mechanical problems persisted. Apprehension grew.

Saturday night, Sept. 18

Today I spoke to Dorothy Bergère and told her of my suspicion—that someone in the crew must be doing all this on purpose & is being paid off by someone to do it (meaning Fr. Casino—but I didn't say). She said yes—that they suspect that and they have "dicks" around everywhere and when they catch that person or persons it'll be awful. She said wires and cables have been cut—*clean cuts that aren't breaks.*

Tonight as we prepared to make our entrance for "Harmony" our stage rolls on and we are in 2 circles, all of us in a back bend on a revolving disc. So half-way out our *stage gets stuck and stops. Bergé says "Quickly go to the floor in front and continue." So, down we clamor and no sooner does everyone get off and down into a circle on the front floor than the stage continues on into its place where it* should *have gone. Funny it got stuck long enough to ruin it all and then 1 minute later it worked* all right. *Well then half the kids loused up the number and the whole thing was a MESS. At the end the bridal procession comes down the MOVING ramp and the thing didn't move—finally it did and started with such a jolt it almost threw them off. They were late getting on to the platform and the fellow closed the curtains before the signal and 4 show girls were left outside of the curtain & had to clamor in. There was such a "stink" made by Sandrini and everyone that the 2nd show went perfectly. And it got such a hand we almost cried with joy.*

The papers (so I hear—I didn't have the money for any cause we didn't get paid) were very lenient and said if that show that was given was just a sample of the one to come—it'll be the most stupendous thing that Broadway has ever seen.

Monday aft., Sept. 20

The last show went perfectly for mechanicals last night. And almost perfectly the first show. We got stuck coming on in the "Harmony" again, but we were on enough to be seen so it didn't make as much of a mess as the night before.

Don Ameche was there last night, last show. We rehearsed the Sun Ballet yesterday aft. From 2 to 6:15. It doesn't go in until Wed. though—when we'll give the entire show.

There's a whispering campaign all over Broadway that the rat is presumably from Fr. Casino, so I think he's getting a little worried. Maybe that "whispering" will worry Fr. Casino too & the dirty work will stop because already their business has been affected and we don't even have the whole show on.

Haven't heard anymore from Joe…

Monday night—late, Sept. 20

Rudy Vallee was there tonight at the dinner show and apparently liked the show very much from his expression & applause!

Rehearsed awfully *hard today & I'm exhausted tonight. One platform ran off the tracks tonight first show and loused up "Harmony", but last show it ran off the tracks again but it got on far enough so it was OK anyhow. We have about 10 different routines to follow—just in case. Never a dull moment!*

Tuesday night, Sept. 21

Tonight when the revolving platform that was removing the dancers who precede us, and our platform was moving on stage, we heard a crash and splintering & knew something had happened on the other platform. We were a wreck all thru our number. Sure enough—as they rolled off a curtain caught on the set and splintered the thing to bits. A stage hand who was on top—behind—got pinned between the scenery that fell and the wall. He wasn't hurt, but got scared skinny—not knowing where everything was going to fall. Naturally it spoiled the whole scene because the bridal procession couldn't come on and the curtain had to close on us. That was the last show. The first show, the whole business went absolutely perfectly *and it just about tore down the house! One of our girls' hats was stolen from the dressing room tonight. And this afternoon when one group of dancers returned to their dressing room after rehearsal, their pants and garter belts all had holes cut out of them. And one of their costumes had been slit 3 inches!*

In the Journal *yesterday it said, "Sabotage was the reason for the 'broken' cable at International Casino on their opening night"—so you see...*

A few days later Peg shares with her older sister, who was

working in Indianapolis, her euphoria over finally being able to add the "Sun Ballet" to the show. Her unbridled excitement completely overshadowed all the suspicious mechanical problems.

Saturday, Sept. 25

Just a note to tell you the good news. We opened a wk ago last night. Last night we did the complete *show for the first time. We've waited 11 weeks to show NY our "Sun Ballet" and, Ruth, they* stood up *and* whistled *and* yelled *and* cheered *and* screamed. *We were all crying. It was the most terrific thing that has* ever *been presented in the WORLD. And, Ruth, that is* not *exaggerated.*

Can you picture this? I hope you can. First there is Dawn—a nude girl facing the back on a high black velvet box. She has 2 black long drapes studded with stars. She holds one end in her hands over her head and 2 fellows dressed in black have the other ends. It's to beautiful, soft music. She just does soft movements and finally the light fades on her as 2 sun bursts appear above. Then 4, then 6, then the whole sun. Then the Sun splits in the center and this big black box opens up and makes gold glittering steps, but high! Another girl & I are the first out—we walk down and there's a HAND and after us come 32 more girls and we fill the steps. We have on gold sequined costumes, completely sequined and small sequined head gears—long gold sequined gauntlet sleeves that come to a big point above the shoulders. The music is terrific. We do our dance and is it ever hard. Oh I just LOVE it. I'm in front thru the whole thing. Even when there are only 2 in front & the lines go back from us. I'm in front of one line & the other girl in front of the other line. We finish the first part and Jeanne Devereau comes out on toe with huge balloons and brings down the house with her number. After that we start the 2nd part with 4 boys doing swell ballet stuff and then we finally finish. After we finish we walk up these long ramps off either side and stand there. The Sun Burst set moves off stage while another set moves on. It's Apollo in a chariot drawn by 4 cellophane horses. Apollo has only a gold G-string on and he has a divine physique. As this takes place, 32 show girls come down out of the ceiling and they have on complete covering tights of silver sequins and wear capes of gold with silver sequins. Then 16 more showgirls walk down the ramp, past us, and they are all the goddesses—what costumes!

When the steps appeared out of the ceiling is when the audience stood up and whistled and yelled. There was just no stop to the miracles *that they were seeing. Oh, Ruth, we were all so happy we stood on those ramps and cried. Mr. Bergé and Sandrini & Charles were almost in tears from happiness too.*

Mechanical problems with the production abated, but all the complicated maneuvers brought occasional challenges, even for the musicians.

Friday night--/(Sat AM), Oct. 1--(2)

Night 'fore last who was in the audience, right at the front railing but Doug Fairbanks, Jr. & a party (4 in all). Tonight Paul Lukas was there. We had packed *houses both shows, jammed to the brim, and the Sun Ballet was SENSATIONAL the last show. We got more applause etc. than ever before. The first show tonight the orchestra got all lost in the music to it* [Sun Ballet]—*it was just too, too sad. The music is 5/4 time and we have to count everything because there's no way of telling what step to what strain. That's the 2nd time the orchestra got lost. They were all drunk I think!*

This "glamorous" life came with a price tag. The regular human chores still had to be done. When you worked until after midnight, it made your "evening" a bit out of sync with the rest of the world.

Sunday aft, Oct. 3

It's so hard to get up in the afternoons, even after 8 hours of sleep! We never get to bed before 5 or 6 AM. When we get home (about 3 or 3:30) there's always something to do besides the regular chores of washing hose, and pants, putting up hair, etc. Last night I washed my hair [no blow dryers in those days] *and had to read all the Sunday papers to see if there was anything in it about us. Every night at 4 AM is letter writing time! I am dead tired after a very strenuous day on not too much sleep and in such sultry weather that I perspire from buttoning up my high polka shoes!*

Tell Mary that Olsen broadcasts from our Casino quite often, maybe every night. He is absolutely the grandest *person, and has personality plus. During the rehearsals when there was so much trouble with the stage, Olsen was in his overalls and dirty shirt, up there with the laborers, hammering and drilling and pushing stages on and off and you'd never believe that it was the celebrated maestro, George Olsen. No matter how much trouble there*

*ever was, he always had a smile. I'll ask him for a picture
for Mary, the first chance I get.*

Peg had now been away from home for over six years, but
her closeness to her family...a pattern that would continue
throughout her life...was apparent in all of her letters.

Wednesday night—late as usual, Oct. 6

*Sunny & I want Betty to come for a visit at
Thanksgiving time. But, I'll write Betty a letter and tell
her all about it. And Mary can come anytime she feels like
it. Daddy too, and you too, Mom. Everybody. The reason I
suggest Thanksgiving for Betty is because my debts will be
diminishing by that time and it'll be better that way.*

*If there was a "rat" maybe they got rid of him. I don't
know. Or maybe he was converted, once it all got going.
At any rate, no more accidents—knock on wood—and
everything is going beautifully. And I thank my Presence
every time I think of it (during the day) that I have such
a wonderful and beautiful job—that isn't a "job," but a
pleasure trip each night.*

Later that same week...

Friday, Oct. 8

Dearest Mary

*Our letters crossed in the mail. Can you come the 5th
or 6th of Nov.? Is that OK? I can't wait till you come and
the Reddy's* [Sunny's parents, where Peg roomed at the
time] *extend a cordial invitation to you and everyone in
the family to visit us. You'll have the time of your sweet life.*

And maybe, if luck is with you, you'll get your picture of Olsen. By the way, when you come here, you'll have to put your age way, way down in case anyone asks you—you're 18 or maybe even 17. What a life—I have to lie so the whole family has to lie!!!

Family news served as a balance for Peg. One foot was in this storybook life she was living, the other connected her to the real world.

Wednesday aft., Nov. 3

Dear Mom—

Your letter and postal just came and oh Mom, when I read it I told Sunny & Jimmy and then burst into tears—of joy! Then I read that no one except the family is to know about it. So they have sworn to secrecy. I'm so thrilled I don't know what to say. I know how happy she [Ruth] must be and how lucky Van is. Oh dear, am I happy for them. I want to be there and as far as I know this show closes sometime in June, so I could only make it then. Anyhow, don't tell Ruth, but I'm going to start making things right away for her. She deserves the best and she's going to get it. Isn't it funny when you're so extremely happy about something or someone, you cry! I can't seem to stop! I'll write her a letter after I get thru with this.

Gee, I can just see Ruth happily situated—making a darling home out in Wyoming. Mrs. Reddy says those fellows out there are the BEST. They just don't come any finer. I'm so thrilled I can't stop thinking about it. And by golly, I won't let her work after she gets married. She's going to be a wife and not a working one either.

In the summer of 1931, before Ruth was summoned home, she found a summer job in Yellowstone Park. There she met and dated a fellow employee from Montana State College. Ray Van Fleet, known to all his friends as Van, became Ruth's favorite date that summer. In the ensuing six years they wrote sporadically but did not see or talk to one another. Ruth never forgot the twinkle in his blue eyes and early in 1937, at her sister Mary's encouragement, she began writing Lt. Van Fleet. He proposed in a letter dated Sunday, October 11.

Peg's excitement over Ruth's engagement was soon tempered by another sister's misfortune.

Friday PM, Nov. 19

First I read Bet's letter and was so glad she got permission to come. Then I read yours and when I came to the end, I could hardly believe what you had there in black & white. That poor kid. Anyhow, I've just written her & I'll send it air mail special to the hospital. I promised her a shopping tour for herself when she comes over the holidays or whenever she can manage to get the time. And tomorrow, I'll send her a pkg. And, I'll write her every day and send her cards.

Hope Mary got rested up all right. I'll bet she was surprised to find out about Bets when she arrived home.

Let me know how everything progresses. How long will Betty be in the hospital?

Be sure to tell me all about Ruth's announcement party.

Betty remembered the incident clearly over 60 years later. "One night at supper time I couldn't eat, and Ruth thought I should get to the doctor. So, Mother and Daddy took me. It was acute appendicitis, and off to the hospital and surgery I went. It was just before Thanksgiving, and I did so want to be home by then. I made it, but it took so long to recover. Ruth was always looking out for me."

A cable sent to the family on Thanksgiving, had added meaning that year.

Today I am thankful for life and for health but most of all for you

Peggy

As the year drew to a close, Peg still found excitement and gratification in the International Casino...especially when she had a chance to "strut her stuff" for her ballet teacher from Cleveland.

Sunday, Dec. 12

Who do you think saw our last show last night? Pop [Mr. Popeloff, Peg's dance teacher from Cleveland] & Loretta Clemens. They hurried back after it and asked for Emily and me. Oh my golly, I was so excited. So we all went to Emily's apt to talk and have a drink. They were crazy about the show. I asked Pop if he was satisfied with my work and he said he's not only satisfied but proud of me!

Pop asked me how Mary was coming with her voice training. So I told him she had to discontinue it due to financial reasons. He said he didn't care for her teacher she had before but he asked me to tell her to come to see him and he'd have her sing for Gladys (his wife) and maybe they

*could do something for her. So Mary, there you are! Get
yourself something worked up and go up and see him.*

Once again Peg would spend the holiday season away
from home. Excitement over her sister's forthcoming marriage
offset the frustration she felt over the unresolved issue of her
own marriage.

***

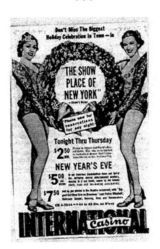

Peg *(r)* ad for
International Casino

DANCING FOR THE KING
1938

The year dawned with the International Casino in full swing. Sabotage efforts which had plagued the show in the Fall of 1937 had disappeared. However, the business climate in show business was beginning to change. Many weeks of rehearsal without pay...dismissal without cause...fluctuating wages. These issues were no longer acceptable. The country's economic climate was improving and workers everywhere were demanding fair treatment. Broadway was no exception. Peg found herself thrust into the role of an organizer for Chorus Equity.

Wednesday aft., Jan. 12, 418 E. 51st St. NYC

The thing with Chorus Equity is coming to a head tonight. There are about 66 chorus girls in our show (dancers & show girls). In order for Equity to have authority to proceed they needed 51% of the girls' signatures. They have 46 signatures and really all they needed was 34. Well, Equity sent the Casino a letter stating that if they didn't send someone to confer and come to terms by Wed. at 6 PM the front of the Casino would be picketed. No strike yet— but picketed. Equity wants jurisdiction over clubs and they should have it. The few items they call for are:

a. $40 a week minimum salary

b.   4 weeks rehearsal at $15 a week

c.   *a 5-day probation period (during which time they may let you go—this means first 5 days of rehearsal for any club)*

d.   *one day a week off with pay*

e.   *no one may be fired or replaced without consent of Equity. In other words, if there's a legitimate reason, OK, but not just to give so & so's girl friend a place. See?*

Well, Sunny and I being Equity members have been dragged into this right up to our neck and of course, it is all very secretive. Getting kids to sign the slips and sneaking them back in your purse and then delivering them to the representative whom we meet every night in Hecto's Cafeteria! Finally, last Monday we had a load of show girls' signatures and I had my purse bulging with them. So I went up to Equity myself with them Monday aft. When I walked into Equity I was ushered into the big head's office, Miss Christie, the new Pres. And when I said I had slips—18 show girls and 1 more dancer, my golly they just bowed and scraped and all but kissed my feet! So now tonight is the night and we are all wondering if there'll be a picket in front. You see, the Musicians Union is in cahoots with us by issuing the order that they are "forbidden to play for any non-union performers" and we are the only non-union in the show. Equity is affiliated with AFA and AF of L.

Let me tell you that Sunny & I have gone thru many a very nervous moment over all this. You know, guilty conscience! If we ever got caught before it all came to a head, it'd be good-bye job. Except that Mr. Hale is very much in favor of it and so Sunny felt a little safer after she found that out. Of course we are 100% in favor or we wouldn't bother with it. But so many clubs are closing and not even paying off. The French Casino first, and now the Hollywood closed and did NOT pay off. Joe Moss had the Hollywood and did that and he is our *boss! Equity requires a 2 weeks bond held by Equity and the club would have to post a 2 weeks closing notice. I'll let you know how it all turns out.*

Newspaper clippings, enclosed in a letter mailed January 18, disclose the following:

"Chorus Equity today won the first skirmish in its battle with Billy Rose...It put back on the payroll petite Barbara Hunter, the chorus girl he fired last Saturday for luring his forty-two Texas beauties into the Chorus Girls' Union, which immediately demanded a raise, union hours and other benefits.

"Chorus Equity Association, won its first contract yesterday in its campaign to organize night club chorus girls. According to a union announcement, the proprietors of the International Casino, agreed to recognize Chorus Equity and negotiate an agreement on Jan. 24 to cover working conditions and wages."

Sunday night, Jan. 16

Friday night when we got paid they asked us to read & sign a paper stating, "I am happy and contented with my work and want no part of Equity. I sign this of my own free will and by no compulsion." It had not been officially stated that Equity had gotten us or not, so we knew nothing. All the kids signed and I stalled as long as I could, hoping something would happen. Finally they called for me to come out and get paid, so I went out and read the thing and asked what it was all about. I said to them that I was happy with my job, my salary was OK, I enjoyed the dances I do but said I've been an Equity member ever since my first job, so how could I sign that I want no part of Equity. The paymaster explained that Equity was trying to get in (of course, we all played dumb) and they just wanted to know if we were happy with conditions as they are. But, he implied that I didn't have to sign if I didn't want to. So I said, "Now, wait a minute. I want to get this straight. It doesn't happen to be that anyone NOT signing this paper will be given her notice, does it?" And he only said, "Well, the whole thing boils down to, are you happy here or are you not, and if you are happy sign & if not don't." But he did not answer my question, get it? I wasn't in the position to be independent. I didn't know if Equity was in yet since we had not yet been notified. If I signed I'd keep my job, but would be signing against my own union. If I didn't sign I'd lose my job no doubt…so I signed. That was during the intermission of the 1st show. After the Finale I came downstairs and learned that a man from Equity was here to speak to the girls & I thought, "Thank God" and so did all the kids. Well, he came in & called all the girls in the entire show together & said, "I have an agreement here signed by Mr. Joe Moss stating the following… And he read to us that within 10 days from today (Fri) a contract & final agreement would be drawn that for 10 days no one could be fired or replaced and that Chorus Equity was recognized by the International Casino as sole bargaining agency for all chorus members, etc, etc, and then said "you are NOW under the protection of Equity. Thank you all."

Of course we were so happy everyone was in tears.

We went out to eat and that was when I called Ruth to say goodbye. [Peg's sister Ruth was leaving Saturday on the train bound for Wyoming, where she would marry and begin her life as Mrs. Raymond Van Fleet, Army Wife Extraordinaire.]

The following day, Saturday, I went to Equity & spoke to the head and put myself on the carpet before they could, about signing against them. She said they understood the whole situation and every signature the Casino got, and every Equity member's signature proves there was compulsion behind it.

Continued Monday evening

Betty arrived OK. She waited to eat with me before the show. I told Bets to get to bed, she must be tired since she had no sleep on the bus. And I'll awaken her when I get home. Tomorrow we'll have lunch at 12 with Marguerite & then go shopping for Betty. That'll be loads of fun. Tomorrow night she'll see the show. Wednesday we'll go to Radio City & see "Snow White & the 7 Dwarfs." Thursday I'll go to the gym and Bets can come & watch. So you see that so far we're pretty well booked up.

I just sent Ruth & Van a wire. They must be married by now. It's 7:40. She said around 6 PM our time.

Bets looks swell but I didn't have much time to talk to her. Guess I'd better close as 15 [minute warning before the curtain] *was just called & I must get ready.*

As February rolled around, Peg was ready to strike out on her own. She found a small studio-apartment at 311 W. 72nd Street. Being able to cook again and have some privacy was exhilarating.

Thursday, Feb. 10

I started this at the club but now I am home in my cute little place. Have just bleached & washed my hair. I love the air coming in my window. We breathe in so much smoke when we work at the club, that when I smell fresh air, I just LOVE it!

We have rehearsal tomorrow at 3:30. You see, they are reinstating the "Conjugation" scene Saturday and we do our Polka in that. I am so glad because the more I do it the better I like it.

The chance to "nest" was short-lived, however. Within a month uncertainty again prevailed.

Thursday, March 10

Things happened fast and furiously last night. This is it. We close April 8—a new show goes in April 12. We go on the road in condensed fashion for 3 months. Bergé Ballet & Hoffman girls will be in the show, but not the Hale girls. (Guess he has something else for them, I think London.) And of course some show girls, but not all. When we come back we rehearse for the new show going in Sept. Bergé is not doing the show until Sept. because he wants only to work with us, "his ballet!" The show going in for the summer will be a much smaller show. So anyhow that means 4 weeks from tonight we close here. At least that's the scoop so far. I'm not one bit worried because they'll keep us working & it'll go big on the road even though it won't have dropping stairs, etc. By the time we close I hope to have $100 in the bank.

PS I'm going to room with Teresa.

Even though the dancers now had a union, it had little effect on all the speculation about the show's future.

Saturday, March 12

We are supposed to find out by tonight what happens. Personally, I think we'll stay here. Last night there were lots of rumors going around. My pals, the stagehands, (they know before anyone else what goes on) take me in a corner & tell me one thing. Then someone else whispers something else that's supposed to be absolutely definite—*but don't tell anyone, etc, etc. It's so funny! We're told by Ava, however, that everything will be decided by tonight.*

Jeanne left yesterday for the Beverly Hills Country Club in Covington, Ky. They'll be there indefinitely. It's a nice job & a very swell-elegant place.

Bye bye for now and I shall keep you posted. The notice says we close April 9 or 10 and the new Spring Edition opens April 16.

The yo-yo continued.

Monday night, March 14

God is so good to me. I am so happy I don't know where to begin so I'll come to the point right away. It was all decided tonight and told to us. The show stays here, as is. We all are kept (the ballet girls) and we still get our same salary. We are the only ones not taking a $5 cut. We run until the end of July, start rehearsing immediately and open the new show in Sept. And the ballet girls will be in the new show.

The yo-yo persisted, but periodic show biz publicity stunts provided some interesting opportunities.

Wednesday, March 16

I just got home (it's 5PM) from having movies, movies and more movies taken! We all had to be in at 1:30 & every newsreel company in existence was there. So, go to the movies steady now because we will be all over the world. It is supposed to be a feet & leg contest so we sat with our shoes and hose off for 3 hours. I about roasted under those lights and sweated my new dress up so much I'm taking it to be cleaned right away.

They actually served us sandwiches and coffee for staying so long! It was very trying but quite interesting. Only one calamity. We had to ride up the escalator sitting down. We all got set and they started it up. Then they started it down, and didn't stop it and we couldn't stand up fast enough so we all piled up at the bottom and one girl got her dress caught in it & ripped. I kind of hurt my ankle (for the moment only) and Teresa got hit in the bust! So I balked & so did Teresa and we wouldn't go up on it anymore. I was scared stiff!

Not surprisingly, the recurring uncertainty about the future led to some introspection about life in show business.

Sunday night, April 3

Once again there is talk of this show going on the road, but it isn't definite yet. I'm so sick of doing the same thing. Never in my life have I ever done the same show, the same dances for so long. We are getting lousy in them too—so mechanical—same thing night in and night out, with never, never, never a night off that I could scream sometimes. But of course when Friday comes around I am always very happy to sign for my pay envelope. Isn't it funny though, how you can feel that way?

I've been summing up show business the last couple of days and tried to figure out why *we work. And I've boiled it down to this—for the love of it! Naturally we work for money, but where is the money we've earned? Gone for debts (accumulated while waiting for a job) to live, to buy clothes because we must look nice & up-to-date, for chiropodists, for hair dressers, and a good lot for make up, etc. So, after 7½ months of a steady job we end up with a hundred and some odd dollars in the bank and hope it's going to last you until the next job comes. If it does, you're lucky enough to start from scratch, if it doesn't you start from debts—and so it goes. So we must do it because we love it and when we get too much of the same thing we don't love it which proves I think, that we are just as human as any other working person who gets one day off a week.*

I guess I'm in a lousy humor tonight to ramble on like this, but I'm so fed up—I'd like to go to China, or maybe South Africa would be better since there's no war there.

Monday night, April 11

It's 5 AM & I've been in bed since 4 and just can't get to sleep. Guess the reason for my insomnia is that Mary Brenner, the wardrobe woman came & stood behind me in the dressing room tonight & said, "Peggy, would you like to go to Paree?" and I saw that look in her eye and then all the kids flocked around her & she said she could 'day dream' if she wanted to & passed it off. So, I got alone with her after the show & asked her what she knew. Sandrini's partner is here to take some people back & she said she saw him point to me when I passed & said about taking me to Paris. But she made me swear not to tell any of the kids. Anyhow I hope she was right. Now I'm all a twit and I wish they'd tell us. She said 6 of us are going. Oh, Mom—I wish they'd tell us & not keep us in suspense.

The most terrible thing happened to me tonight during the first show. There was cotton under my feet for the Sun Ballet (there generally is cotton or big kitchen matches from the previous act) & I slipped on it in the fancy turns. Well I got so lost I couldn't get back into the dance and just had to stand still for it seemed ages. When I got off I cried and cried and I went up & told Dupont. Charles was there with him & had seen it. So Jacque Charles put his arms around me & laughed & he said "Never mind Peggy—that's the first time I see you go wrong in 4 years." They were all so nice about it.

I guess the Page boy got bawled out cause he's supposed to clean it up before we get on. I wouldn't mind but I'm front center!!! It was clean as anything the 2nd show!

Wednesday night, April 13

Such news here's a note to tell you. Tonight I was asked to go to Paris in Sept. For Sandrini. I accepted— 900 francs a week which is 225 fr more than we got at Paramount. Oh Mom, God is really good to me. I'm on my honor not to tell anyone here. Four of us were asked. Ava is cabling Sandrini right now that we accepted. She received a cable from him today saying to ask us.

Several days later Peg sends a quick card home saying,

Just a hurried note. Am so excited I can't even eat. Going to Paris in June. Contracts on the way.

Tuesday, April 26

I think we sail June 7 on the Isle de France. Of course we had to keep it absolutely secret. But it got out and by Sunday I was almost losing my mind, lying to all the kids who came & asked for me. Finally I went to Ava & told her evidently everyone knew—how I don't know—but asked her what to do about it. So she said we could tell the truth now. In 5 minutes it was all over the Casino and our lives weren't worth 2 cents and still aren't. I never heard tell of such jealousy. It makes me sick to my stomach. Being mopey & furious & gossipy won't get them a contract now, *and just shows what they're made of.*

Watch the papers every day for pictures of me for the NY World's Fair 1939. I'm riding on the Sports Float next Sat. at the preview of the World's Fair, celebrating one year until it opens. The pictures were taken yesterday afternoon, for 3 syndicates, and will be sent to every Cleveland paper. We ride with Babe Ruth, Gene Tunney and a lot of other sports figures.

On April 30, 1938, Peg rode that float with Babe Ruth! He gave her a cardboard baseball which he autographed in pencil. More than 50 years later she sold it to a collector for $500 and was informed it would have been worth a lot more if it had been signed in ink.

That same day, Peg did her final show at the International Casino. The following week, after contracts for Paris arrived by boat and were signed, she left to join her friend, Jeanne, at the

Beverly Hills Country Club in Newport, Kentucky. The club, across the river from Cincinnati, Ohio was a celebrated night club and casino and a popular stop for famous entertainers. It provided a great chance to earn additional money before heading to Paris.

Beverly Hills Country Club burned to the ground, May 28, 1977.

Thursday, May 5

Leave tonight for Ky by bus. I'll be there 3 weeks and then I go to Cleveland for a week. Signed my contract on Tuesday for Paris. Contract starts June 15 so I guess we sail June 7. We find out later.

My contract is for "6 months or longer," pays 900 francs a week, rehearsal period being half salary, to work at Bal Tabarin or Moulin Rouge. Sandrini owns both places. But Moulin Rouge doesn't open until Oct so we'll be at the Tabarin all summer.

Sunday, May 8 Beverly Hills Country Club, KY

Arrived Friday night and started rehearsing yesterday. It is the MOST GORGEOUS place—way out in the country with cows and horses & fresh air & fields, etc. I can hardly believe it. The air intoxicates me. I'm not used to it. Oh it's wonderful.

Friday, May 13

I've done my first show and now I'm ready for the second. But the second show is all different from the first. The numbers are pretty tough. The first dance in the 1st show is "Josephine" a tap dance in long chartreuse chiffon gowns. The second dance is a German Waltz in peasant dresses and we have trays and pass out real honest to goodness bottles of beer. Then when we get rid of the beer (to the right count in the music) we do a dance with the trays—finally putting the trays down & finishing to "Oh Katherina." The Finale is in long silver gowns, like evening dresses—and we start out with long net capes that have a train. It's done to "Stranger in Paris" & we have lots of just arm movements interspersed with lyrics. Then we take off the capes and do a ballet-ish dance in high heels! Then after all that we stay on and do small stuff while the principals come out. The second show the opening is a tap dance to "Bojangles" in short black velvet costumes. I feel just like Fred Astaire! Oh yes! The next dance is darling, but a headache. It's "Lilac Time" & we each have an arbor of lilacs and we have troubles holding those on each side as well as your own while you dance in and out and all around. The costumes are orchid flare skirts, street length, that look like bedroom curtains. The jacket is green organdie with a flounce on the bottom & lilacs at the waist where it connects in front. And little orchid straw poke bonnet hats. It's awfully pretty on the floor.

Working in Kentucky came with some hazards.

Wednesday, May 18

Night before last they tried to blow up the bridge at the entrance to the club. It shook the place but they must have been amateurs because no damage was done. It was in headlines the next day and it has hurt business already. People are afraid the place itself will be the next target. There were 29 in the audience last night!

But Peg's real concerns were over conditions far from

Newport, Kentucky. The growing political tensions in Europe begin to cast a pall over the upcoming adventure.

Monday, May 23

You know, with Germany so close to war with Czechoslovakia & France being tied into it with a pact with the Czechs, I wonder if they'll still have us go over. I sure don't want to go where there is any war, but why the devil can't Hitler be satisfied with having gotten Austria & let there be peace. Of course if they won't let us go, I'm not going to be disappointed, because whatever happens is for the best. I'll only be sore I put out about $11.50 on a passport!

Cleveland Plain Dealer, Sunday, June 12, 1938

"Peggy Morrison, Cleveland dancer, is sailing this week for her second European engagement. She has signed a contract to appear at the Bal Tabarin Club in Paris for six months. Later she will appear for another six months at Paris Moulin Rouge with three other American girls."

The passport investment paid off. Peg arrived in Paris June 18, 1938 and moved, along with the other two American dancers, into an apartment at 49 Rue Poncelet. Rehearsals for Bal Tabarin commenced immediately.

A month later, on July 20, Peg was asked to join a select troupe to perform for England's King George VI and Queen Elizabeth who were making a State visit to France.

This very special performance took place under sunny Paris skies at Bagatelle in Bois de Boulogne. The Bois is to Paris what Central Park is to New York City.

More than 60 years later, Peg vividly recalled the day. "There were 19 of us. We danced without any music, just using the rhythm of the poetry, to a piece called 'Poesie.' Another number, 'Harmonie,' was performed with music. Both numbers were ballet, choreographed by Marcel Bergé. Our costumes were of soft flowing fabric that wrapped itself around the body just right.

"The 'Harmonie' costume was pale blue satin, full length with long sleeves. The 'Poesie' costume was white, also full length, but sleeveless. We danced to the rhythm of the poetry, read by Frenchmen...in French...which to me, is music!

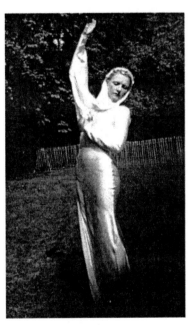

Rehearsing for the King
July 20, 1938

***

"The stage floated in the middle of a lily pond, a la

Monet at Giverney. The backdrop was this enormous boulder, behind which, was 'backstage.' The Royal party was seated in front of the lily pond. In '93 when Carol {Peg's daughter} and I returned to Paris, I tried and tried to find that lily pond. I finally located the big boulder and then realized that all the rest had been especially created for the King & Queen of England! What a shock."

This account from the Parisian magazine *L' Illustration*, July 1938

"The Laughter and Play in Bagatelle"

"...A charming show of exquisite dances performed on a stage in the middle of the little lake made beautiful reflections in the water. The dances symbolized Harmony, Elegance, Fantasy & Poetry. Young ladies in transparent costumes were graceful and sometimes acrobatic. In all an exquisite hour and a lovely venture of romanticism and modernity. Something which doesn't happen often, very distinguished and extremely successful."

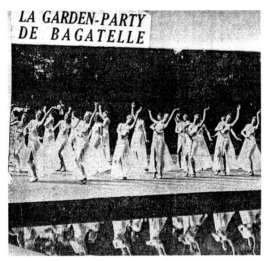

Peg front row 2nd from left
Performing "Poesie"

***

The King and Queen returned to England and Peg's life returned to Bal Tabarin. Rehearsals and performances still consumed most of the dancers' time. However, during their time-off, Peg and her American friends had great fun renewing old friendships and exploring Paris and the French countryside with the young Frenchmen she had met in '33...Rene, Roger & Cupid (Hubert). In a letter to her sister, Betty, Peg recounted some particulars of summer in Paris.

Friday, Aug. 5

Paris is absolutely flooded with Americans & many foreigners, while all Parisians have fled to seashores and the country to get away from this stifling heat. Shops close & have signs "closed for the month of Aug." So no matter where you go, you see & hear Americans. It's wonderful!

Am studying French now every day, out of my Fr. Grammar, learning new words and reviewing construction. I'm not so timid now.

Yesterday afternoon I saw my first movie here. Went over to the Courcelles and saw "Bringing up Baby" and "Breakfast for Two." Yes, they have double features here too. All for 8 francs—about 22 cents—and all in English.

All week long we've not had any rehearsal. Gee it's just wonderful. It's bad enough just doing my 3 little numbers at night in this heat. And the Tabarin is not air conditioned. You can't begin to imagine how hot it is in there. It's always so jammed full of people. I don't know how they stand it. Of course, at this time of year they are mostly all Americans & tourists and they stand anything because Tabarin is THE place to go!

By the time the Morrison household received her letter, they had probably seen the following newspaper coverage.

Cleveland Plain Dealer, Friday, August 12, 1938

"Perhaps a few Clevelanders who saw the news reels at local movie houses last week recognized a familiar face.

"I refer to the pictures of the gala entertainment of their British majesties in Paris recently. At one of the parties a group of dancing girls cavorted for their special delight on a stage set in the middle of a lily pond.

"If you look closely at the girls, you'll be able to pick out Peggy Morrison, a Cleveland dancer and former Popeloff pupil, who is now dancing at the Bal Tabarin in Paris and was chosen for the lucky group who brought pleased smiles to the faces of King George and Queen Elizabeth."

"In those days," Peg remembered, "there were theaters just for news. No TV, you know. Anyway, Mother and Daddy would go downtown and sit all day in the news theater and watch the footage on the visit to France by the British Royals. There was superb coverage of it and they could follow me all through it, all day long."

The glow of the summer's Royal visit must have faded quickly, as the political tension on the Continent continued to mount. As oblivious as everyone seemed to be, issues in Europe were heating up and the talk of war escalated. On September 26, Peg received an official communiqué from the American Embassy in Paris advising her, "If your business in France is not critical, you should prepare to return to the United States."

Peg and her American roommates informed the Embassy they were under a contract they could not yet break.

Three days later, September 29, 1938, the Munich Agreement, signed by Germany, France, Italy and Great Britain, gave Germany the Sudetenland region of Czechoslovakia. It was an effort by the European powers to pacify Hitler. The American Embassy offered United States citizens the chance to move to the Embassy, so in the event war did break out, they would be on American soil. Again, Peg and her American colleagues declined.

That autumn, dancers at Bal Tabarin learned of a new ballet forming for the Scala Theater in Berlin. Some dancers were asked to submit a photo to the German government in order to be considered for this prestigious opportunity. Peg hopefully submitted the required documents, but was turned down. The German government erroneously suspected this blond, fair-skinned dancer was Jewish. A couple of her friends, however, did go to Berlin as part of that new ballet.

As she had done for several years, Peg augmented her income with odd modeling jobs.

***

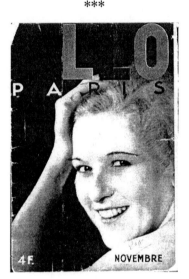

Paris cover girl

***

On November 8, a young Polish Jew, Hershel Grynszpan, assassinated an official at the German Embassy in Paris. Young Grynszpan acted out his frustration over his parents' expulsion, along with 15,000 other Jews, from Germany back to their native Poland. Young Nazis across Germany responded with two days and nights of violence, known forever after as "Kristallnacht," "night of broken glass." Over 100 synagogues and 7500 Jewish-owned businesses were destroyed and some

26,000 Jews were arrested and sent away to concentration camps.

Less than a week later, Peg made an abrupt decision to return to the United States. Her crumbled marriage to Joe Ancona, her ever-present financial struggles, and a growing awareness of political sickness spreading across Europe, fueled her decision.

> *Sunday night, Nov. 13*
>
> *Have just made up my mind to quit Jan. 15 and come home the first boat after that. Have it all figured out—and am I ever happy! The way I figure is this. I'm absolutely wasting time here. I can't get a divorce here, the dollar keeps going up, and now our income tax has gone up from 50 francs a week to 91 fr a week on account of war preparations & the government money used for it. So, we foreigners have to help pay. By Jan. 15, I figure I can put enough aside to go home on. Haven't been able to save one penny yet.*
>
> *I'll just take a chance on getting a job when I get back. Maybe it won't be a dead season. Maybe it will. But I'll try my luck. I want to go back. I've weighed the good & bad on both sides of the Atlantic & reasons why I want to stay & why I want to leave & I really think I won't be unhappy. Yes, I'll hate to leave Paris itself because it is* one beautiful city. *And I'll hate to leave a very beautiful language behind. But I shan't be sorry to leave Tabarin, or the filth and degeneracy and sex that hang out all over the night life. I'll be sorry to leave behind my wonderful friends here too.*
>
> *Wednesday we are having tea at Anna's home. She's the little French girl in our dressing room. Actually, she is*

not French, they are Polish. I asked her if they couldn't take citizenship papers here. They've lived in Paris 15 years. She said that 5 years ago they tried. Her mother didn't understand the word "oldest child" in a question—it is an expression very French, that would not be understood except by someone really educated in France. They were refused papers. The following year they applied again and were refused this 2nd time because their children consist of 4 girls and 1 boy, instead of 4 boys & 1 girl. One boy is not sufficient in the family for future wars! Nice work, eh! They applied a third time the next year (2 years ago) & haven't heard from them yet. She said that if they had 5000 francs to slip the fellow, they could be naturalized without any questions or anything. Isn't that terrible?

Saturday, Nov. 26

I am sailing for home Jan. 4. I just can't stand this Tabarin anymore. Figured that by squeezing every centime I could leave Jan. 4 & I spoke to Sandrini today. He ok'd it & will arrange my ticket etc. It is on the S/S Paris, the boat you saw me sail away on my first trip here. I'll arrive in NY January 11.

I want to start my divorce immediately. I looked at all angles, and I feel it is a waste of time to stay here any longer. I want to get my divorce, and I want to get out of this business. I think 7½ years is enough.

Now that I've given my notice I wouldn't stay any longer. I don't want to. But the dirty louses are making me rehearse for the new show even though I am leaving way before this one finishes. Just to be spiteful—they are full of *those tricks because they are sore that they can't make me stay.*

So this year, in which the world was undergoing irrevocable changes, closed with Peg preparing to leave France.

ESCAPING THE WAR
1939

And leave she did. Leaving the accelerating crisis in Europe behind, as well as friends and colleagues, Peg sailed into New York Harbor in early January. The voyage was a rough one, filled with winter weather and rough seas. Trunks were tied to the wall so they would not fly around the cabins. The ship was filled with people who had left Europe due to the brewing war. In Peg's mind, their arrival in New York seemed very dramatic. "I at least expected the Marine Band to be on the dock playing the Star Spangled Banner," she recalled. The New York Port Authority was oblivious to the high emotions of the passengers. Their arrival was treated as just another ship coming in to port.

Friday, Jan. 13 New York City

...Before I left Paris Mr. Sandrini told me to let him know about 15 days or a month before I'd be free here, if I wanted to come back. He is counting on my returning in about 3 or 4 months. Which, of course, is very nice as who knows what might happen.

Following a job with Simmons Tours, performing on a cruise ship to the Bahamas, Peg joined a Chester Hale-group rehearsing the can-can. Once the act was perfected, they expected to book with the highest bidder.

Sunday, March 26

...On Friday we got paid for the job Tuesday night—5 bucks. I spoke to Hale at the same time & asked how much longer it'd be until we started to work. Said I understood it took us this long to get ourselves into shape & learn the tricks, etc. He said he'd know about something in about 3 or 4 days and we wouldn't rehearse more than 2 wks more. Tomorrow we are to start learning the waltz. Now that we have lost our soreness we can "go to town."

Saturday, April 1

Go Mon. or Tues. for costumes. But still don't know where we're going. Wish he'd tell us. It's awfully embarrassing to say to my friends for 3 weeks that I don't know what I'm rehearsing for! They'll soon think I'm crazy.

Particulars of the job remained a mystery.

Thursday, April 13

Well, tomorrow Georgie Jessel is coming in at 4 to see us do our stuff. Apparently they've decided the money and he wants to see us. We don't have a rehearsal today, but I am going in anyhow to limber up and practice a little. I didn't do a good walk-over yesterday so I want to work on that too.

The following day:

The big news is that Georgie Jessel and his manager came today to see our Can-Can and went absolutely mad *about us. Gee, we were wonderful, if I do say it. And my*

*jumping splits were absolutely colossal! The kids said I was
so high up off the floor & was already in a splits when I
was* in the air! *My kicks were positively smack straight
up to my shoulders. Oh it was just wonderful. Monday we
will know definitely. It is not a B'way show. It is "Little
Old NY Village" at the Fair* [1939 World's Fair]. *If we
get it, we will start rehearsing Tues for it, because we'll
have to learn more numbers. It opens May 15th, but after
1 week of rehearsals we get rehearsal money, which is, I
think, $15 a week.*

*If something goes wrong that we don't get it, there are
several others who are clamoring for us. Guess word has
gotten around that Hale has some sensational Can-Can
dancers. Oh yes, if we get it, it's a 22 or 26 week contract.
Keep your fingers crossed. Monday night I'll send you an air
mail so you should hear Tuesday one way or the other. Gee,
I wish it was Monday already.*

Happily, the troupe did get the job at the Fair.

Friday, May 19

*...Sunday we start rehearsing at the Fair, and have
publicity pictures made. Wed is our first dress rehearsal
(full salary starts) and on Friday we give one show at
night to the public. Saturday is our official opening to Gov.
Lehman, Mayor LaGuardia, Grover Whelen, etc....Eddie
Cantor is going to be in our show at the beginning.*

Once the show opened the schedule was grueling.

Sunday, May 28

*Yesterday we opened to the public at 6:30 PM with a
parade. At 7:30 we did a show, at 8:30 another, next at*

10, then 11:15 and last one at 1 AM. That was 5! They had over 20,000 in the Village and they were going crazy clamoring for shows. Eddie Cantor, Gracie Allen & George Burns were guest artists. They appeared twice....We were so exhausted. We didn't even have time out to eat. It was practically one change after another. And Can-Can until unconscious. Today we do 12 shows (6 Can-Cans).

Throughout all these years, the issue of Peg's divorce from Joe had never been resolved. They had not lived together for over three years, but all efforts to terminate the union legally had been for naught. Within weeks after the excitement of opening at the Fair, there was once more cause for hope.

> *Friday, June 9*
>
> *I'm so excited I can hardly write, so this is just a note to tell you that Patsy* [fellow dancer and former roommate] *rec'd a letter from Joe's attorney asking my whereabouts. I guess he's getting a divorce!! I'm going to see my lawyer tomorrow and get some legal information on it. Will let you know as it goes along.*

> *Tuesday, June 20*
>
> *Just rec'd a registered letter advising me " I beg to advise you that a meeting to take testimony in the above named matter will take place in my office on Monday, July 10, 1939 at 3:30 PM (DST)" Ref. Ancona vs Ancona."*
>
> *Will see a lawyer now.*

While the legal wheels ground along at their customary slow speed, work at the Fair continued to be fun. In addition to dancing, Peg had her first, and only, comedy role.

Sunday, June 25

Big news! Your daughter has become an actress. Yes, I do a "bit" with Jack Goldie, and it's the best laugh in the show. He says he's going to do some impersonations. First is "Dracula" and he puts on a hideous fake face and makes awful noises, etc. I walk out, look at him, very straight faced, and I'm not at all scared. He goes through much stuff to try to scare me and then he says "Oh, what the hell" and takes the false face off. I look at him and give with a TERRIFIC scream and fly off the stage. Gee what a laugh it gets! And, I just love to do it. He was going to let different ones do it, but I'm so good (he says) that the part is mine! Isn't that exciting?

The divorce saga continued.

Monday, July 3

…Patsy got that information for me. I must have a representative in Phila. on July 10 or the divorce will only be legal in PA. So, I'm seeing the lawyer Wed. and he has a friend who is a lawyer in the same bldg as Joe's lawyer in Phila[delphia] who could represent me. It'll cost me something, I don't know how much, but I've got to do it.

As often happened, a happy event emerged in the midst of Peg's grueling schedule and the grinding divorce bureaucracy. In 1931, Peg's family had befriended a young man, Bill Plambeck, from Hamburg, Germany. Bill had studied at Case Institute of Technology for a year, and had been a frequent visitor to the Morrison household. He had dated Peg's sister, Ruth, and helped Mary with her French. Bill had returned to Hamburg following his studies, but maintained his contact with the family. In June of 1939, Bill was in New York on business, and looked Peg up at the Fair.

Wednesday, July 5

I'm sorry I've kept neglecting to write about Bill's visit. He came in during the Finale of the 1st show and ordered dinner—alone, and sent back word with a waiter that he was there. Since we aren't allowed to sit with friends I went out and explained it to him and we sneaked a little chat right there. He said he was sorry he couldn't ask me to dinner because he didn't have enough money. He could leave Germany with only $22 and he didn't have much left! Poor kid. He looked just grand. *We made a date for outside the stage door after the fireworks were over and I had about 25 minutes to spend with him. We went over and got 2 bottles of coca-cola and sat down on a bench in front of the Hall of Music and talked and reminisced. Half the stuff I couldn't even remember, but I said "yes" to everything. He sure remembers every minute of the good times he spent with the Morrisons.*

I tried to get him to say something about Germany, etc, but nary a word came out. They must be scared to open their mouths. That was on Thurs. He sailed on Sat. So I asked him to have lunch with me at the Belgium Pavillion the next day (we were invited to bring a guest in payment for dancing there) but he was too busy and couldn't do it. So we parted at 11 PM and he about shook my arm off and said to be sure to be remembered to everyone. The doorman kids me yet about the "German Count" who took my arm away with him!

The "house rules" that prevented Peg from joining Bill's

table when he visited the Fair were enforced to protect the dancers and preserve the integrity of the Village.

Sunday, July 16

...I don't know if I ever told you how we can't look *at a man or come in smelling of a drink, or anything—at Old New York Village. We call it Georgie Jessel's Reform School! We aren't allowed to sit with friends, we aren't allowed in the Village, we can't do anything!*

As the summer wore on, so did the divorce proceedings.

Wednesday, Aug. 2

...Went down and paid the lawyer some more money today. (I now only owe $30 more—isn't that wonderful?) He informed me that the 1st or 2nd week in September I will receive my final *divorce papers and according to PA law, my name can automatically go back to Morrison if I so wish. Since the divorce will be granted in PA, my name of Morrison will also be legal here or anywhere else. Isn't this all swell news?* [Morrison had been her stage name all along.]

Summer's end also brought news of the worsening situation in Europe. The friends and colleagues, who remained in Europe, were much on her mind.

Thursday, Aug. 24

...Now I'm so busy reading the papers that it's awful. I guess René is already called because they called in "3" and "4" and he's in "3." Bergé and Sandrini are in "5." [Reference to the French draft system which took the lower numbers first.]

The kids, Lee & Doris [the American dancers who

had stayed behind in Paris] *are supposed to sail for home a week from today. I wonder what'll happen. Everyone here seems to think it* will *happen. But I just can't believe it. It's worse than last Sept. I guess. Had an air mail from the kids, mailed Sat., I got it Tues AM, but no mention. Of course it wasn't "hot" last Sat. like now. Well, I'm sending them an air mail today. It doesn't leave till Sat and they'll get it Mon., if they get it at all.*

Thursday, Aug, 31

It's 3:30 AM or so, and I've been listening to the radio. Golly it sounds like it's really started. Air raids, etc. British fleet rushing to Poland—Godfrey! Isn't it terrible? Doris & Lee are supposed to sail tomorrow (Fri). I hope they do. I wish I'd hear from René. He's been gone (to the frontier somewhere) over a week, but of course, I guess he can't write. Must get to bed so I can get up early & find out about the war.

The following day, Sept. 1, 1939, Hitler invaded Poland. World War II had begun in Europe. That night the following radio report came out of Paris. "The two American girls dancing at Bal Tabarin sailed for home today on the S/S Manhattan." Peg's friend, Sue, who had gone to dance in Berlin, was due to sail for home September 14.

Sunday, Sept. 3

...Of course the only subject—or about the only one— for talk is this terrible and unwanted war. I just can not believe that it has actually come to this point. Of course all my friends are in it, and I guess Bill Plambeck is too.

[Bill Plambeck was required to serve in Hitler's

Army. Twenty years after his meeting with Peg, Bill was reunited with Peg's sister, Ruth. Bill shared with her some of his wartime experiences. He said that toward the end of the war, when it was apparent the Germans were going to lose, he started carrying a suit of civilian clothes with him at all times. He knew that when the Americans arrived, he didn't want to be in a German uniform!]

...The S/S Athenia which was torpedoed and sunk tonight is sure a crime. According to one report I heard a Cleveland person & 9 year-old son were on it along with countless other Americans.

The Queen Mary is expected to dock in NY sometime tonight and has a convoy of 2 battleships. I wish the S/S Manhattan would hurry and get to NY ahead of time. Mr. Hale [producer of Peg's show at the New York World's Fair] *has a troupe of 12 girls in Cannes. That at present isn't a danger zone, but they could quickly scoot to Italy as long as they remain neutral. And personally, I don't think that will be long. I heard Deladier speak this aft. And also Roosevelt tonight. R. couldn't really say very much more than he did, do you think? After all, we are neutral and he couldn't give any personal opinions or say much more than to declare our position as neutral and to advise people against believing rumor, etc. I don't really know an awful lot about war, or what the delicate intricacies are in regard to outside nations, so I can't be a good judge. But, he made me feel proud of the USA and proud to be an American.*

Of course, I have no word what-so-ever from René. If I do, I'll let you know at once. I'm going to write to Mr.

Sasso, Roger's father, and ask him how I can get word to René. He may know if I can even get a letter to him, or he may have left Paris too for the outskirts.

Incidentally, I heard tonight a recorded broadcast as picked up by short wave. It was from the government controlled broadcasting station in Berlin, and was a report of the news, in English. Well—we were almost hysterical it was really so funny—actually funny! Weird stories of how "the Poles have persecuted the Germans for ages and how the poor German people never put a harmful finger upon the Polish people. How Hitler had sent the message of 16 points to Britain & Poland and sat and waited 48 long hours for a Polish representative to come, so he was forced to protect his people by meeting force with force, since the silence from both countries meant they were warring with him! Everything *is Chamberlain's fault, and Chamberlain is a crook and a horrible person who has thrown his nation (Germany) and also his own (England) into a war. Poor Germany strived to every possible means to keep peace but England wanted war. England is ALL to blame." A very fancy bit of news. I'd say! Try to listen to one of those. Your hair will stand on end!*

Though the atrocities raged across the Atlantic, everyday life in the US went on pretty much as usual. Tiring of the World's Fair routine, Peg was on the lookout for another job. This time, however, the look was short.

Wednesday, Oct. 4

I'm so excited & nervous I can hardly write. Just auditioned for Radio City Rockettes and was taken! I can open Oct. 19. Oh, he liked me so much! You're supposed to

*do a chorus of tap (4 steps) and I didn't even finish the 2nd
step & he said "Fine"------Oh, golly, I could just shout!!*

Founded in 1925 by Russell Markert, the Rockettes were,
and still are, the quintessential American chorus line. They
marry precision drill with great style. The troupe opened at
New York's Radio City Music Hall in 1932 and the next year
began a format that continues today…a new show with every
new movie opening. In those days, that was weekly, as a rule.
Through the years the Rockettes have awed audiences all over
the world.

Peg had landed the job most dancers only dream of.

Thursday, Oct. 5

*I told Stanley tonight that I could open at Music Hall
with the Rockettes 2 weeks from today & explained it all to
him. He was just swell about it. I told him I didn't want
any hard feelings because I didn't have any, etc, etc. Well,
he thinks that no matter what I do, it is OK. Said he just
knew I'd go over there & as much as said he didn't blame
me.*

*As you already know, yesterday was a big day. Tap
lesson 1 to 2 PM, acrobatic 2 to 3 and then I practiced
until 3:30. Then over for the audition at 4. That in itself
made me a nervous wreck. Then we did 4 shows last night
for the first time in 3 days.*

There was time for fun, though. Even time to try
something new.

*Recently Charlie & I went out to Bethpage & played
18 holes of golf. I can't even cough in peace now! My ribs
ache—my arms ache & my hands are so I could hardly*

crush a feather!! I'm going to take a few lessons and get some pointers on the game. Then, maybe I can stop swinging and missing*!! Teeing off for the first hole & always a few people standing around—you get all prepared, step up to the ball, get your eye glued on it, swing that club in such beautiful form (you think), and son-of-a-gun—after all that, the doggone ball is still sitting there on the tee just as pretty and unmarred as it was before!! So, you try again, this time it connects, but something funny happened because instead of the ball traveling about 100 yards toward the first hole, it lands 3 feet in* back *of where you're starting!! By that time you turn around and mutter a "tough hole, eh?" And you finally land the ball in the proper direction—even if it is only 25 yards off! Some fun huh?*

Remuneration from the Rockettes was the best Peg had seen in over eight years in show business.

Wednesday, Oct. 25

Got my first check tonight and it looks so nice. It says $41.58. That's with 42 cents off for Social Security. I'm going to get my rings out of hock tomorrow too. That'll be $4 plus interest.

Finally, news from France.

Thursday, Nov. 2

This morning I rec'd a letter from Roger. He wrote it Oct 5—today is Nov. 2! My letter to him took a month too and he answered immediately. Well, he gave me René's address, and also Cupid's [another friend from Paris]. *René is not fighting—thank goodness. He's an instructor in Saumur. That's where he rec'd his military training. So anyhow I know he's safer than if he were "up the line."*

The ever-changing venue at Radio City left the Rockettes almost constantly preparing for a new show. Their show changed with each new movie shown at the Music Hall. Some movies played only a week, others two, and very rarely, some even longer. The longer the show ran, the more challenges the dancers had keeping their routine fresh.

Sunday, Nov. 5

...next we do 2 numbers. For one the costumes are one-legged pajamas. One has a leg and the other leg is bare. Oh boy, no kicking with the wrong leg!!! The other number is "Bolero," done with the ballet. Because we're working with the ballet too we'll also have to rehearse nights between last 2 shows. But I don't mind. Can you imagine the pleasure of dancing to such beautiful music as Ravel's Bolero?

Wasn't that just wonderful that I rec'd a letter from Roger all about René & Cupid. I wrote all 3 of them air mail letters. Gee I was so happy to get word of them. I could have cried for joy.

Sue Harris [a friend from Bal Tabrarin who had gone to dance in Berlin when Peg had been rejected by German officials, suspected of being Jewish] *is apparently lost. Her family is frantic. Washington DC has even tried to find her, but no luck. The American Embassies in Germany don't know where she is. No one knows. Oh isn't that just awful? A friend of hers here rec'd a letter written in German stating that a letter to her from Sue*

Harris had been taken by the censors. I guess it was written by censors. Isn't that awful?

Thankfully though, Sue survived her harrowing experience.

Thanksgiving 1939 Nov. 23

Sue Harris came around to see me the other day. Ye Gods! Here's the story. She'd gone to a very swanky party with a Count. It was the day before Czechoslovakia was taken. Of course everyone was discussing it and the Count said there couldn't be a war because Hitler was such a dirty dog some one would shoot him first. Well, one thing led to another and a lot of the people started damning him (H). The next day the Gestapo came after Sue. They kept her for 4 hours, questioning her about conversations that had passed and what had been said about their "god." She didn't let a thing out. Explained that she couldn't understand German well enough to get anything, that she could understand if the person was speaking directly to her, and spoke simple German very slowly. But, she never heard anyone call H. a "dirty dog." In the meantime, this Count was put into a concentration camp. He was kept there 8 weeks. And for 8 weeks Sue was trailed by a Gestapo agent. No matter where she went, he trailed her. Well, 2 nights before she was supposed to sail she was invited to another party, all people from her theater. She decided not to go, and good for her she didn't, because the next day the Gestapo rounded up everyone who was there and no one has seen hide nor hair of them since.

Sue had written a letter to her mother telling her not to worry, she was OK, didn't know her plans as yet, etc.

The only thing she mentioned that might have been censored was about not getting very much to eat and the ration cards, but she spoke of it very joyfully with no offense whatsoever. Her mother received the envelope, but no letter.

She had German money for her passage and of course, no one would take it. That's what held up her getting home. She finally got to Norway or somewhere and managed to get enough money for her passage and got on the boat with $2 American money!

I sure do have plenty to be thankful for.

Charlie left $5 for Virginia & me to have Thanksgiving dinner. So, we had our dinner yesterday, since she left for vacation today. We went to Longchamps—one of the snootiest and most expensive places. We couldn't get turkey, but we had chicken. Our dinner consisted of tomato juice, roasted boned baby chicken, little potatoes, green peas, cranberry & apple sauce, & coffee. It came to $5.04!! Can you imagine such extravagance!

The fabled Rockettes Christmas Show opened at Radio City Thanksgiving weekend. It was a turning point for Peg.

Friday, Nov. 24

...Set a record for myself yesterday. Opening day and I ate lunch and also dinner. Wasn't nervous, at least not like before. Naturally, I was a little nervous, but didn't get those flip flops in my stomach and that feeling just before the opening show that I'd have to quit. So that's really something.

Sunday, Dec. 3

Emily told me tonight I get my vacation the week of Dec. 14. Can you imagine me having a whole week off and getting paid $42 for it? I just can't believe it.

In her eight-plus years in show business, that was Peg's first paid vacation! That wasn't the only good news to come her way that month. Her six-year marriage to Joe Ancona finally came to an end.

Friday, Dec. 8

How did you like my telegram tonight? Wanted to say "On the loose again. Love from your divorced daughter, Peggy" but I sent it from the theater so I couldn't. I'm so relieved it's finally over.

The first really good boner was pulled in the March last night. And wouldn't it have to happen to the girl next to me! She has been making mistakes all week but this was really the prize. It was when we all are at the footlights and every other girl turns around and marches up the elevators 22 counts while the other girls remain standing still at the footlights. After we get up to the top on 22 and "about face" on 23-24, the others who are still down stage "about face" and do what we just did while we march on down and we cross thru each other. We get to the boots when they get to the top and we all turn around and go back and everyone meets in 1 straight line in the middle of the stage.

Well, I go up stage first so that means Margo & Muriel stay there and just wait 22 counts. But Margo marched up with us and it wasn't until about the count of 5 that she realized she was wrong. She started to go back and then changed her mind and went all the way up with us. Then we go back down while the others are coming up and instead of just hopping into her place as the 2 lines crossed thru, she came way further down and then decided to run back up stage and join them. It was a MESS!

Yet another holiday season away from home loomed. But life was good. Peg returned from a week's vacation, she loved being a Rockette, even doing five shows a day, she'd had good news from her French friends, and all her American colleagues were home safely. A year ago she had hastily prepared to leave France as the nightmare that became WW II unfolded. Now, in December of 1939, her mood was quite the opposite.

Friday, Dec. 22

Already I have 5 gifts staring me in the face at home. The trouble is that I don't know when to open them. It's no fun opening them alone on Xmas Eve. And to bring them over here on Xmas day would be almost impossible because I have to carry over 16 packages for theater gifts and they're no small easy ones to handle. Then if I waited till Virginia got home Xmas night, Xmas would be all over. Isn't it wonderful that a thing like that is my biggest problem at present?

Never have been without a tree and we weren't going to have one this year cause we'd be so busy with 5 shows a day. But yesterday I broke down & got a little one and trimmed it last night. It's all blue & silver. We have it on the mantle. Gee it's so pretty.

Guess this is all. Sure wish I could be home with you for the holidays, but I'm getting so used to it now it would probably seem funny and too wonderful to be true.

Wednesday, Dec. 27

Yesterday we rehearsed at 7:15 AM to 10:45. First show 11:15. Lunch & a shower, second show, rehearsal, 3rd show, dinner, 4th show, preview, 5th show. Then home & to bed by 12:30. Up at 6 AM today, rehearsal 7:30. Five shows again, rehearsals between. Tomorrow rehearsal at 7:15, 5 shows & rehearsals between. Then a midnight rehearsal after last show. Friday no rehearsals. Saturday Dec 30 is opening day [of the New Year's Show] *so dress rehearsals at 6:45 & of course, 5 shows, also 5 Sunday & 5 Monday. I feel like I've been drunk for two months. Remember everyone said how tough it was here at Xmas time? Well, it sure is. But I don't mind.*

An eventful year drew to a close. One marked by an abrupt and prudent exit from France. She left behind a continent now ravaged by war. Close friends were in real peril. The lengthy and difficult divorce proceedings were finally over. And Peg was now a member of an elite and prestigious sorority. More than 60 years later her bond with the Rockettes is still strong.

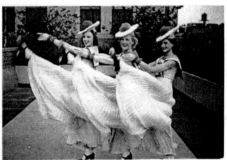

Rockettes rehearse rooftop, Radio City
l to r Virginia Henry, Peg, Diane Parris

LIFE AS A ROCKETTE
1940

Life as a Rockette brought subtle, but important lifestyle changes. For the first time in her career, Peg had a job with a perpetual run. A sense of job security she had never before experienced. The financial pressures that had haunted her over the years were now a thing of the past. She was regularly able to send money to help her family, take some nice vacations, and generally enjoy a life free from worry over how to pay the rent.

New routines kept the Rockettes fresh and challenged. With new shows generally every week, life was a continuous round of performances and rehearsals, but they loved it.

The novelty of paid vacations continued to amaze Peg.

Wednesday eve., Jan. 31

Say, isn't it something, me getting a "2 weeker?" I work 2 weeks and I'm off again! That's because I worked that extra week before in order to do the tap number.

Now sit down, or get a glass of cold water and prepare for something really nice. A wonderful surprise. I'm coming home for my next vacation. And when is that? One week from tonight, I will leave at 11:40 PM and arrive in Cleveland at 11:22 AM on Thurs. I can stay until Sunday, but I think I'll have to leave Sun. morning

*to get back and have a good sleep to start rehearsing Mon.
at 9 AM.*

*The funniest thing happened this last show today, and
it happened to ME! I forgot to zip my pants. The costume is
short black velvet. I am in the front line! And we do several
steps turning around where it would show just terribly.
And I wondered why the drummer was laughing so hard!
Oh dear. I didn't feel it or know what the funny breeze was
until the last line up of kicks and when I realized what it
was I could have collapsed! And when the curtain came
down and I told the kids the whole place was in hysterics.
They had me doing the different steps etc to see how much it
showed. I about died! I shall be most uncomfortable looking
at the musicians next show!*

*I'm starting at Berlitz tonight taking French. I've
wanted to for oh so long.*

Sunday aft., Feb. 25

*Filled out and mailed my income tax report last night.
A man comes to the theater and does it for you and tells you
what you can put for exemptions. He listed mine as:*

Make up, etc.	*$50.00*
Rehearsal clothes/shoes	*50.00*
Chiropodist	*50.00*
Cleaning/laundry	*52.00*
Church/charity	*20.00*
Sales/admission tax	*20.00*

*That much from my total earnings for 1939 brought
me just under my $1000. Assisting in the support of a*

family does NOT count. It only counts if you are the "head" of a family and can claim a dependent. ...Next year, if I'm still here, I'll have around $2200 I think, and that's plenty to pay tax on.

That man notarized both reports, State & Fed., 50 cents for both. I'm glad it's off my hands now.

Stability also meant better accommodations.

Friday, March 8

Virginia and I are moving this Sunday to the following address—Belevedere Hotel W. 48th St. NYC. We have a one-room apt, which consists of a lovely room with bath & kitchenette, all for the same money we pay here. We will have a PRIVATE bath. That is the main reason for the move.

Today I received a letter from Roger [a Parisian friend]. *Says René is promoted to Lieutenant and is "somewhere in France" and has left Saumur where he was teaching. Of course, that's an advancement but I don't like it as well as him being an instructor.*

Peg's love of the French language continued to inspire her. Weekly lessons were a priority for her, in spite of often being exhausted from performances and rehearsals. She found stimulation and sometimes "comic relief."

Wednesday night, April 3

Here's something funny that happened in French class Monday night. I kept yawning, so the teacher made me conjugate the verb "bayer" (to yawn) the whole way through in the present, past, future and the subjunctive (we are on

139

the subjunctive now). Gee we had a good laugh about that! By the time I got through everyone including himself, was yawning!

We're doing such a terrific business [Rockettes] *that passes can't be used over the weekend! It'll surely be a 3 weeker, and I'm hoping it'll be 4. I'd be off the 3rd week of it and come back to the same number. That would really be something.*

Peg's divorce presented opportunity for a new kind of social life. Platonic friendships had defined her relationships with men during the years of her marriage to Joe Ancona, even though they had lived apart. Finally, she gave herself permission to look at men in a new way.

Thursday Night, April 18

I've met a man! A French man! He is one of the most interesting persons I've met in ages and ages. His name is Bernard Lamotte and he's one of the best known artists in France. He does 3 magazines here, paintings, sketches, illustrations, etc., for Fortune, Life and Time. He speaks practically no English, and so, of course, I speak French every minute I'm with him. I'd say he's in his early 30's but I'm a bum judge of ages. I hope, I hope, I hope he stays nice and that I don't have any of the usual difficulties because I'd really like to see a lot of him. He doesn't give me any heart palpitations, but I just like his personality—and manners—and conversation, etc. He can speak so intelligently on practically any subject. Last night he showed us the proofs of 8 pages of paintings for Fortune. They were mostly of war-time Paris and one just made me ill! It was Notre Dame all barricaded with sand bags!

What gorgeous work he does! Oh yes, I met him through my French teacher. Had dinner tonight with him and also a fast night lunch. Bernard gave me a ticket to a private exhibition of his paintings at the Fine Arts Museum, Penthouse Gallery or something.

Thursday night, April 25

The other night Pierre, the Fr. Teacher, and Florence, Bernard, my Fr. Artist friend, and I and Russell Markert [Rockettes founder and choreographer] *went out. First we went to the Casino Russe and then to La Martinique. I had the most marvelous time. Well, in the course of the evening I had the most glorious dance in my life. It was with Russell Markert and we did Rumba and Conga for at least 20 minutes. At first I was petrified. But not for long. He gets terribly fancy, and everyone knew who he was so everyone was watching. He leads so beautifully you just can't help but follow, no matter how fancy he gets. It was the first time I'd ever done "ballroom" Conga!! I've done it on the stage but it's sort of different.*

PS Forgot before to tell you most of the Rockettes, including yours truly, are knitting sweaters for the Red Cross (for flood sufferers).

As a result of Peg's French studies, an idea began to germinate.

Friday night, April 26

Something funny happened tonight that I must write to you about. And it's strange too that you just mentioned it in your last letter. You suggested using my time and energy to prepare myself for some other sort of work instead of studying French. Tonight I had another French lesson. In the course of it, he had us each translate into English some passages from stories. He explained that to translate is VERY difficult because one must be sure to keep the same tenses of verbs, yet change into another language exactly *what the author has portrayed, not in a sense of making it literal, but still making it comprehensible to the readers of the 2nd language, not losing or adding from or to the original. When it came my turn it was a little story we had never studied before. We read it through and any words we didn't understand he explained (but all explanations are in Fr.). Then I started. It is something I've never done because when I read Fr or speak it, I think it, and don't translate, so I was a bit leery! When I finished he was flabbergasted and said that as well as he knew both French & English, I did 100% better job than he could do! (Incidentally, he doesn't hand out compliments on a silver platter). Then he started on what I want to write you about. He said that any time I was tired of dancing I could easily get a job doing just that* [translating]. *He told us of all the different fields there are for it, and that just when he started his new school he was offered a job at $75 a week with an oil company to translate French & Spanish into English. And, he kept on talking and talking about it until it really sunk in as an excellent idea. Magazines, newspapers, radio, commercial companies, etc., are only some of the fields for it, and that it pays at least $50 or $60 a week.*

So now, what do you think of that? I just love French and I'd love to take up Spanish again. He didn't mention the Spanish, but of course, in a line like that, the more you know, the better.

I've been thinking about it ever since, and I honestly think it was an idea "sent" to me.

Cont'd next day.

Talked to Betty & Freddy Roberts til 2:30 A.M. Hadn't seen them since one day in Deauville. They were in Biarritz when the war started, finally got into Italy and from there went to Buenos Aires and Rio. Just got back a couple of weeks ago. Gee we talked and talked and talked. Such funny stories about the war. They were almost arrested for being spies! When Freddy explained the whole thing, the cop who came to get them sat down and had laughs and drinks with them! They are a dance team. She was in our troupe at the Paramount in Paris and met Freddy in Biarritz when we were there. Since then they've worked in the same shows and finally got married.

Guess I'll sign off now and do some French. One show down, 4 to go!

Unlike the chat with Betty and Freddy, news from her French friends caused Peg more anguish than laughs.

Wednesday night, May 22

Today I received a letter from Roger (in France). It was mailed April 15. Nice & long and interesting. He's still training. Says René was appointed to a Regiment but didn't know which and was being given training for the General's Food Staff "something like a glorified headwaiter" as Roger puts it. So, I hope that means he's only a staff member and not carrying a gun!

Guess I'd better sign off and get to bed so I can go over the new routine a few times. That's where I get good practice—thinking it through in bed.

As mentioned, new routines were practically weekly events. By this time, Peg had opening-show jitters under control, and most openings went smoothly...but not always.

Thursday night, May 30

Today was opening day, besides being Decoration {now known as Memorial} *Day and 5 shows. So for dress rehearsal we got up at 5:45 AM. We work in the ballet too and there is only 6½ to change from that into our number. It is just terrible. Our costume is in 6 pieces, consisting of socks, then gaiters (leggings) which zip up—then you put on your tap shoes and fasten their straps, after that, you fasten the gaiter strap under the shoe!!! Then you get into your costume and pants (2 pieces). They both zip from bottom to top up the back. Besides that you have 10 snaps and 7 hooks and eyes plus sleeve zippers. Then you put on your hat and then your gloves and you have 2 hooks and eyes on each glove to fasten them to the sleeves so they don't come down. If you can picture getting into all that garbage in 6½ minutes and being able to remember the routine afterwards—well you're a better guy than I am! Our dance is just wonderful, although it's a corker and you can get "off" just as easy as that. I made a beautiful mistake first show. But there were so many that it didn't matter.*

Tuesday, June 4

...Am enclosing the last letter from Roger. I rec'd it 2 weeks ago tomorrow. Thought you might like to read it. You see, I had asked him if I sent a couple of dollars if it would get through OK. So the first part of the letter is in answer to that. Would you please send it back to me. Oh yes, I crossed out 2 places that are slightly off-color and thought

you'd prefer not to read those words. They weren't awful,
but just better not read.

Isn't the war just terrible. I get sick to think that
Paris is bombed. How can it be? And now LeHavre—I
just can't believe it.

The social consciousness fostered among these young
women was amazing. Contrary to the stereotypical image of the
self-centered, egotistical, entertainer, the Rockettes frequently
did benefit performances and took up worthy causes. Most of
them had performed, at one time or another, in Europe, and
had personal concerns about wartime events.

Friday night, June 7

Today a woman came to the theater—she went over
to Paris with the Rockettes in '37. She's French, was just
a passenger on the ship, but everyone liked her and she and
her husband taught the kids French every day and helped
make their trip a pleasant one. Now she's one of the heads
of the American-French Relief and the kids [Rockettes]
are going to help them. We just got through knitting for
the Red Cross so no one wants to knit. So, we will fold
and wind bandages, sew and bring in old clothes we don't
want. I've just rounded up old dead clothes I never wear
and also 4 pair of shoes. I ransacked 2 dresses, 2 sweaters,
a blouse, a skirt, 2 heavy pair of gloves, a pair of pjs, a pair
of gabardine slacks and a set of woolies. The kids in the
dressing room save lumps of sugar left over from coffee they
bring in. We have about 7 lbs. That's going too. Tomorrow
the woman is bringing over the bandages, etc, to show us
how it's to be done. Any money that is donated is spent in
the US and the merchandise sent across. Naturally, I want

to do all I can so I am pleased that I can find clothes and shoes to give them. And, of course, I'll sew and do bandages too. She said the refugees pouring into France haven't even a handkerchief to their name. They have no shoes and as makeshift ones, they sew together layers and layers of newspaper and tie it around their feet. Honestly, it just makes me ill to think of it.

Well, I told Mary [Peg's youngest sister] *I just had a feeling something would prevent all of us from going to the Ranch in Sept* [a planned vacation]. *It has started. At least if we go we can't go into Mexico. No one can leave the US or cross a border without a passport! So, they are going to have a big revolution in Mexico in July and heaven knows what it'll lead to. Personally, I think the US is getting in deeper and deeper every day and I can't see that they can help it. After all, if Hitler takes over Europe, he'll surely head for the Americans, so if we don't help the Allies now we'll have an even worse job on our hands later on. Not that I'm in favor of wars, but I sure am patriotic enough to want us to defend our country and that demon should be stopped before he goes much further. A Senator claims Hitler is already at war with South America and the US since he's sent his 5th column ahead and they are now operating. So why shouldn't we aid the Allies in supplies and materials, whatever we can. I don't know much about wars or anything like that, but that's the way I figure it out!*

Wednesday night, June 19
...Last night I dreamed Hitler had taken over the USA and I saw him and his pot-belly marching down 5th

Ave. or somewhere and anyhow I was crying so hard it woke me up and I was weeping something terrific!

Tuesday night, June 25

…That's a wonderful idea sending those clothes to the relief. Yes, I guess they are still taking things but they make sure that they don't get into German hands. If necessary, they'll send them to England.

Incidentally, they caught that notorious "Peggy Morrison" the day after they interviewed me. We sure had a laugh about it. I think that's the strangest thing that ever happened to me.

It was so strange, in fact, that sixty years later Peg vividly recalled the incident. "One morning I got up early to go shopping. Virginia (her roommate) met me at the theater and when I arrived she told me she had something to tell me, and that I'd probably better sit down. She said she'd had a phone call from some man in the lobby of the hotel (we were living at the Hotel Belevedere). He said he had to talk to her about her roommate, Peggy Morrison. Virginia got dressed and went down to the lobby. The man told her he knew I'd gone shopping. He was from the FBI. He was after a "Peggy Morrison." He knew I was NOT the one he was looking for but there was *another* Peggy Morrison living in that hotel. Prior to this, late, late at night, after shows, I'd be doing laundry, writing letters, and I'd get a phone call from some man who'd go on and on about all these good times we'd had. I had no idea who he was or what he was talking about! I had 2 or 3 of those calls. The FBI man told Virginia this other Peggy Morrison was from Detroit and she was wanted for prostitution, drug abuse, etc. He knew I was a different Peggy Morrison, but he had to interview me anyway. He knew *everything* about me. He told Virginia he'd give any future husband of mine a good reference, cause he knew I'd always left my dates in the lobby and never had one come upstairs! I was to show him my passport for verification of who I was. I immediately told Russell Markert before he got it through the gossip mill. Before I could go collect my passport, they caught the *other* Peggy Morrison and the whole thing was over!"

Our Peggy Morrison continued her routine of performances, rehearsals, language lessons and work for the American-French Relief Agency. In May she had augmented her French studies with Spanish lessons, resurrecting a language she hadn't used since Argentina in '36.

With rediscovered fluency in Spanish, Peg and Virginia decided to vacation that September in Havana. They sailed down on the S/S Oriente and spent an idyllic week at the Hotel Nacional.

October brought long-awaited word from France.

Wednesday night, Oct 9

Will enclose a copy I made for you of a letter I received this Mon., Oct 7, from Roger. You'll notice I left out some swear words, marked the space like this xxxx.

The envelope had been opened and the sticker pasting it closed is marked "opened by examiner 1492," but I'm sure that had it been read, it never would have gotten through.

August 8, 1940

Dearest Peggy,

How to begin this letter is a problem to me. After all

that happened in this poor country, almost any news that I can give you will be about 6 weeks old by the time I write it, and much older still by the time you get it. First of all, let me answer a few questions you are sure to ask. René is alive and uninjured. He came out of Belgium via Dunkirk, fought in Normandy again, near Evreuce, and I know he is in perfect health just now though I don't know where. I got a post card from him dated July 19, but he gave no address, and I was therefore unable to answer. Hubert [their mutual friend, Cupid] *is also alive. I'll tell you later in this letter how I knew it. He also went through Belgium and Dunkirk.*

As for me, the story is shorter. I was in Saumur, as well you know, and was scheduled to be an officer on July 10. Instead of which, orders came on July 15 that courses were to be stopped and we were to be turned into a fighting unit. On the 16th and 17th we were armed and equipped as best they could. Well, all we had was rifles and machine guns, no artillery, not even anti-tank, and as far as equipment, a tent cloth, a bandage to dress a wound in case of emergency and 2 day's rations.

On the 18th we left Saumur and were camped out in a farm, where we stayed one night, and we heard and saw the bridges on the Loire fly up in the air, on the 19th we moved, and at 3AM on the 20th, bombing and shelling began. At 5:30AM we got orders to go on the banks of the Loire, to prevent the Germans from crossing the river. We piled 30 of us into 2 cars, with all our belongings and ammunition, and before we got half-way from the river, we discovered the Germans had already passed, and were shooting at us. So we stopped the cars, got out of them, and started to fight. But, this we learned later, and were damn proud of it, while there were only 165 of us cadets fighting in that place, there was a whole German division—anything between 3 to 5000—I mean 5 thousand men against us with light and heavy and anti-tank artillery, aviation and mortars, besides while we had a rifle with 45 cartridges, every man on the other side had a submachine gun, lighter than our rifles, shooting about 500 rounds per minute, with a practically unlimited reserve of ammunition. We had our "fusil mitraelleur," a light machine gun, heavier than a rifle, though weighs about 23 lbs, a marvelous weapon, but too heavy to be handled like a submachine which weighs about 7 or 8 lbs, but much more accurate. Still, as is normal in the French army, one out of 10 of us had one, and while it can shoot 450 rounds per minute, we had only 250 cartridges for each.

Nevertheless we resisted more than 8 hrs, and even threw the Germans back by a few hundred meters, and then the order came to abandon our positions. When we had a roll call, we found out of my platoon of 30, 12 were missing, and out of 165 in the squadron, only 90 answered the call of their names. We knew later there had been 17 killed, the rest more or less seriously injured.

Then we drove away, about 10 miles, and found out we only had 40 cartridges left for 18 rifles, and 150 for 4 light machine guns. We got orders to reach a village called Lerné, 25 miles away, stopped for 3 hours in the woods to rest and played hide and seek with the Germans from 6 PM till nightfall when we finally found a free road to reach Lerné.

There we waited from 5 till 8 AM on the 21st and

the orders we got were rather surprising. Throw away your arms and surrender when the enemy turns up. They were orders and therefore not to be discussed, nevertheless a mutiny almost broke out. All the more so since our colonel said, "I am the soul of the school, and I shall get away while you are taken prisoners." Old xxxx.

At least they did not have my rifle. I took it to bits, scattered the pieces in a nearby forest, threw the barrel in a pond, and broke the butt to splinters. Then rather sad, feeling more like having a good cry than anything else, and being very very dirty and tired to top it all, I proceeded towards a farm to have a wash and a shave. While shaving, I heard a booming voice shouting my name, almost cut myself to death at the sound of it, and turned around to find Hubert! He and what was left of his regiment had landed there and the next day at 11 AM we were taken prisoners together.

That was June 22nd, and from that day, until July 6 when we were freed, we walked 400 kms. Together, stopping 3 days at the most in the same place, covering 30 miles on the worst of our strolls, after which his regiment went one way, and my school the other. But while I don't know what's become of him, this is a brief account of our doings. We spent a fortnight in a combination mill and farm, lying in the straw or hay all day. Then a 20 kms walk to a village which is the border between the occupied and non-occupied areas, where we were to take delivery of 780 horses, the whole of the Saumur stables, including all the finest show prizewinners which had been caught by the Germans while they were being taken down to Montauban, in the SW of France. The horses were to be freed, but the men with them were to be kept prisoners. So the 780 horses for 200 of us.

While we were supposed to sleep in the straw, a few of us found better lodgings. With a friend of mine we found a huge room with 2 beds, as we had not seen one in ages. And you may never have seen a French peasant's bed. It is a huge affair with curtains hanging all around it, springs underneath, 2 feather mattresses, sheets and blankets of course, and an tremendous, bright red feather eiderdown. We slept in them for 5 days, and no horses came. Then we were switched somewhere else, and the 780 horses we saw all right, but their riders were there too. But they were demobilized after 2 days and at last we took charge of the beasts. And then, for a week we belonged to the horse: at 7 AM take them to drink, brush them, and take care of them, (which includes in the French army, washing the animals eyes and backside and genital organs with a sponge every other day); at 10, drink, feed; at 2 PM drink & ride; at 5 PM drink, feed and brush. I had 2 of the xxxxs. One, a boy, is about the tallest horse I ever saw and its name was Dragon II. The other was black, and I was not on very good terms with it. You see, Dragon was only a biter, and with a good punch on the nostrils, you kept him quiet for a while. As for the other, he was both a biter and a kicker. So, when you punched him he kicked, and when you beat him he bit. So xxxx to it. I lent it to a friend of mine to ride one day, and he was thrown 5 minutes later. As for Dragon, I discovered too late, he was a jumper, and anything from the shadow of a tree up to a ditch or a hedge was something to go over, and that however hard you tried to hold him back. I can't understand why he did not throw me. But I am rid of horses now.

We got them into a train. You know, whose box cars we have in France. Well, in my group, 100 of us embarked 300 of them. Started at 7 PM one day, and finished at 1 AM, with the beasts scared by the lights, and the darkness of the cars and what not, and we rode 400 kms with them, talking to them from 1 AM on Aug 1st till 6 PM on Aug 3rd, bouncing out to give them to drink as soon as the train stopped. All I know is we were dead when we arrived, and then we had to feed them once more, and brush them before we got them into their stables by noon. And we had to start work again at 2 PM, feeding etc. I think one of the luxuries I'll seek after the war is never seeing a horse again!

Finally, we were relieved of the horses, and taken to a Godforsaken village called Nohie, in the Southwest of France, 10 miles from Montauban, which is quite large and where the horses have beautiful lodgings.

As for us, we are divided and lodged in cowsheds, which is good enough for a human being. But in 4 days time, I'll be a civilian again. Yet I can't go back to Paris, or rather don't want to go back there at once, for it is occupied. Besides, my family is in St Jean de Luz, which is also occupied, and I can't get in touch with them. So if you feel like dropping me a line, I'll be at my aunt's and here is the address in Castelnaudary. It is in the south, not very far from the Pyrenees, or from the Mediterranean. Somewhere around Toulouse and Carcassonnne.

Please give my love to everybody we both know.

Love, and unless you object, kisses,

Roger

The importance of this eloquent report from her friend in the thick of the war, was evidenced by the fact that Peg hand-copied this lengthy letter so she could share it with her family and still feel close to Roger by holding on to his letter. But the war was still far away and New York City life continued to be full of diversions.

Peg's steady income afforded her the opportunity to accomplish something new...save some money. She knew, realistically, she couldn't dance forever, and was working toward a "nest egg" for the future. She sent her dad $10 each month, which he put into her savings account. That was in addition to the $15 she sent to help her family with household expenses. In spite of regular pay checks, it was necessary to manage her money carefully.

Saturday eve., Oct. 19

Had a nice visit with Auntie Clyde. We had dinner together and she treated. Wasn't that nice? Especially since I've budgeted myself so strictly. I allow myself 20 cents breakfast, 40 cents dinner, and 20 cents night lunch, so now I'm a little ahead. Of course, on rehearsal days I stick in another 20 cents for lunch. That gives me plenty to eat without squandering anything. I just eat at the places where I can get more for my money!

Peg's command of languages continued to be an asset.

Saturday night, Oct. 26

...Last night there were 50 Army officers from every country in Latin & South America, standing in the wings watching our number. As you know, we are doing a military tap and drill, and gee you just should have seen our number that show. I never saw such a flawless performance! There

wasn't even a nose or a finger or a hair out of line! When the curtain came down they swarmed on stage and Mr. Van Schmuss (mgr of Music Hall) introduced everyone collectively and because I'd been to South America & Cuba, I was ushered to this man and I got a chance to strut my Spanish! ...The man I spoke to mostly was quite old. His name is General Penso (I think) from San Salvador.

Several of the Rockettes took up an interesting hobby that fall...colorizing pictures. Enhancing the black and white photos of the day, gave them a touch of realism, which was fairly rare for the amateur photographer.

Sunday night, Oct 27

...Yes, all those pictures are for you. Now about how to color them. The picture must be printed on dull paper (not "glossy") and I have a set of a certain kind of oil paints that are for that purpose. It requires only a little practice but if you make a mistake you can take off what part you want to with something called "extender." It's like, or rather the results are like, it was an eraser, but it looks just like a tube of Vaseline.

Peg's post-divorce freedom brought some interesting men into her life. One can only imagine the appeal these dancers, with their world-famous legs, had to eligible (and probably some not so eligible) men. One can also imagine the feelings most families had when their sons brought home girlfriends in show business!

Wednesday night, Nov. 6 [written during vacation]

From time to time I've been dating a fellow—he's alright, but far from putting any throb into my heart. His name is Harry Jewett. I don't know how old he is, but figure he's around 34—he's my height—has very little hair (!)

Sunday we drove up to Nyack, NY where his yacht is in dry dock for the winter and he showed it to me and made arrangements for all the repairs, etc. It's 28' long, has a nice sized cabin with 2 double bunks, a stove, ice box, a "johnnie," etc. The deck out in back is quite large.

Yesterday being election day, he didn't have to work. He asked me to have dinner at his home. He lives in Short Hills, NJ, quite a ways from here. I knew his family must be wealthy, but oh boy—what I went through yesterday! We went out by train and he stopped off to vote as soon as we got there. The line was long and finally his mother & father came out, having finished voting (for Wilkie). I was introduced, and they suggested I go on home with them because it'd take over an hour for Harry to go through. So I did. Their home is simply beautiful. Of course, it is HUGE—but the grounds I guess cover about an acre. There is the greenhouse, the rose garden, the this garden and the that garden, a pretty little pool (in the garden, but not a swimming pool). Well the place is just the last word. Dr. Jewett took me all around. I think he's a dr. of science or something—anyhow it's not an MD or a dentist or the like. I believe he's an archeologist—and pray tell what might that be? Study of stones? He's for one thing, a trustee of the Carnegie Foundation. Oh yes, the family car is a Packard limousine. "Charles" is the colored butler, chauffeur, etc. "Sally," his wife, is the cook, maid, etc.

Dinner was served at 7 and oh it was so good, but so darned stiff and stilted! Can't you just see papa at the head *and mama at the other end of the table. Harry on one side, and me sitting on the other side opposite him!! Papa carving a roast chicken that was so big and beautiful it didn't look real—and "Charles" serving! I was ravenously hungry, but I had to act like a lady! It was really funny. Then came chocolate pie for dessert and it was so good I could have eaten another piece, but of course, it wasn't suggested and had it been I would have gracefully declined!*

We talked of Europe and South American and they told me about Japan. They've been everywhere. After dinner we had "coffee in the drawing room"(!) and then they brought out the projector and we saw my color films and many, many of theirs, from their last trip, which was to Guatemala. …It was very *interesting.*

Harry & I left about 9:30 to come back to NY. We stopped for a drink at some place nearby and we got to NY about 12. Had something to eat downstairs here and listened to the election returns till 1:30. In the meantime he's telling me how much he likes me, etc and backed it up by saying, "why do you think I ever asked you for this date today—to meet my parents!" He's hardly even kissed me! A couple of times he's "pecked" me on the side of the face!

He's a perfect gentleman—inclined to brag a bit I'd say, but he's very intelligent & well-bred. For the time being I guess I'll go out with him when he asks me, but the whole thing yesterday had me a little in a dither—mostly when he said he'd purposely asked me out for his parents to meet me & visa a versa.

Peg continued to enjoy the ever-changing routines and resulting challenges to her talent.

Sunday night, Nov. 24

I just LOVE the dance we do this week. Am so glad it's holding over because I'm off next week and I can see it from front & take some good pictures. It's a Scotch Highland Fling. I've never done one before. Gosh I wish you could see this—it's just wonderful. We get a hand about 4 different places in it. That's how good it is!!

Every so often though, the dancers were humbled.

Thursday night, Dec. 12

The March went so badly last show, we have a rehearsal at 9:15 tonight. That's pretty soon now. You see, today 10 vacation girls came back to work and so many of us had our places changed and really the lines have been AWFUL all day. You get used to a "pace" (how fast to walk) and then when your place is changed you have to also change your "pace" in all the "wheels." So, no one is used to it and oh, it's been terrible.

Charlie, Virginia, & I are going to have sandwiches and a little party in our room on Xmas Eve & open our presents together. I think he'll get a kick out of that. I remember last year he opened his presents in his car in the parking lot! I felt so sorry for him but you see, Virginia wasn't here & I just didn't want to take him to my room at night when no one else would be there. Altho' there'd be nothing to be afraid of where Charlie is concerned, but it doesn't look good & I don't do it. So, since Virginia will be here this year, we'll have a little party.

Sunday night, Dec. 22

The Xmas show opened Thurs. with much jitters. I

don't know when I've felt so unsure of a number. But we came thru with a perfect score thank goodness. The show is just darling. Kids just love it. The ballet does the Old Woman in the Shoe. The Glee Club boys are snowmen. Then there are some precious marionettes—usually I don't like that kind of act, but gee these are simply marvelous! Then we come on & we are dolls, Yankee Doodle ones with George Washington wigs & hats & cute costumes. It's a cute number & funny in parts and gets good laughs.

Hope you all have a wonderful *Xmas…*

By now the Rockettes' holiday schedule was old hat to Peg. Doing five shows a day, celebrating Christmas with friends, and also at the theater, dulled the ache of yet another holiday season away from home.

***

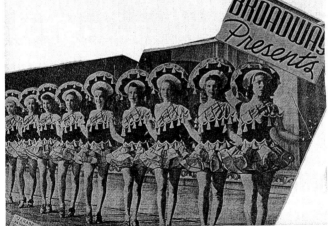

Rockette line Peg, 5th from right

SWEPT OFF HER FEET
1941

Januany brought the familiar round of performances and rehearsals.

> *Sunday eve, Jan. 19*
>
> *The show is being held over for a 5th week. Now it is equal to "Snow White" for the number of weeks. If it stays after that it'll equal "Rebecca." So far it has the attendance record. Gee it sure is a good picture. Be sure you see it—"Philadelphia Story."*
>
> *Only trouble with such a long run is that we do such a stinking number & besides that we do Bolero with the ballet. Our number is over 5 minutes long (that's VERY long) and Bolero is about 10 minutes of jumps!*
>
> *Did I tell you I had a letter from Cupid [Hubert]. He went thru Dunkerque —was sunk in the Channel & in the water some time before being saved! He's the one who Roger met in that farmhouse & they were taken prisoners together. But, he says altho' he's free now & a civilian "it is not all over yet & we may soon be back at work." He's in un-occupied France.*

Hubert's letter to Peg was dated 23 Dec. 1940

> *My dear Peggy*
>
> *It seems fantastic to receive a word from you. I did*

not know Roger had given you my address so it was such a surprise. Many wishes for a happy Xmas (you will get them too late), but lots of happy wishes for a happy New Year too.

Did Roger tell you how we met in jail last June? Jail, I'd better say as prisoners, but as we did fight decently, the Jerries were decent too and we received the Honors of War and set free after a couple of weeks.

It really was an extraordinary adventure. We fighted [sic] *twenty days in Belgium, then lived the whole drama of Dunkerque on our way to England, we were sunk in the Chanel* [sic]*…No fun such kind of bathing and at last were saved, joined and went through England. We then were shipped back to France (submarine chassed* [sic] *and everything) and went back to fight at Saumur with the cadets. I met Roger there, and there too the armistice met us. I'm a civilian again, but the whole thing is not over and it might not be long before we go back to "work."*

You will excuse my English which is not so good. I'm completely out of training…

The Rockettes' management understood that in order to keep their dancers fresh and always at peak performance, they needed frequent breaks from the grueling schedule of multiple performances (up to five) every day, plus almost constant rehearsals. Although there were generally 36 in the line, there were actually 46 on the payroll, ten of whom were on vacation at any given time. Dancers generally performed for four weeks and then had a week off with pay. Frequently they had to be available for rehearsals or costume fittings on those off weeks, but they didn't have to perform. Once or twice a year the dancers were given 3-4 weeks off for extended vacations. The first week was paid, but the others were without pay. Illness and injury sometimes upset the delicate balance of scheduled vacations.

Friday night, Jan. 24

...There are 7 girls out and I do NOT get my extra time off this month. She said I could probably have it next month. Last Tuesday Olga broke her ankle! She'll be out at least 4 months. There are 3 cases of flu! Wow!, a sprained ankle, an appendectomy, a tonsillectomy & 2 vacations of extra time granted from some time back. Those 2 would be called back to work but they are un-reachable! For 2 days we've worked with 35 & Emily, our line captain. I should get my regular week off next week. If it turns out that I don't have time to come home, I'm going to tell everyone I am, so I can have my time selfishly to myself. You may think I'm stingy with my time, but honestly, my friends are too generous & too nice to me. They all know when I'm off & I get invitations from one end of Jersey to the other end of south Brooklyn! And if I accepted them all I'd be ready for a rest sanitarium! By the time I do all my personal chores which mount while I'm working, then I want to do nothing but whatever I feel like. Maybe it's old age. Or maybe it is plain selfishness. All I know is that 24 hours isn't long enough to accomplish all I'd like to do in one day.

It was a time of patriotic fervor in America. The war in Europe and the tragedies being endured by France and England, left most Americans feeling an emotional tie to their ancestral homeland. As one of the premiere symbols of the United States entertainment industry, the Rockettes often did routines that made a political statement of support for the Allies.

Monday night, Feb. 10

It's all mixed up why the show might be held over. The picture is changing for sure. The title of the stage show is "The Last Time I Saw Paris" featuring the popular song by the same name. The Glee Club sings a French military song and then, through a scrim they are seen marching through the Arc de Triomph & they're singing "La Marseillaise", [the French national anthem]. *It gets a terrific hand. Then on this same scrim they show the Rockettes leaving for Paris in 1937, in Paris on the steps of the Opera, and finally the actual performance at the Grand Palais with the huge staircase behind them. They show a good deal of a kick routine and the girls are in one line doing a step with a lot of "knee-ups" when the lites go on behind the scrim, the pictures (newsreels) fade out and then we are discovered on a huge staircase like at the Grand Palais and we are doing "knee-ups" and dance and kick and knee up down the 20 steps. It's really terrific! Well, the French people of something or other, or maybe the French Gov't here, has requested that the show be held.*

Peg was continually becoming aware of war-time trials and tribulations of people she had known throughout her career.

Thursday night, Feb. 13

...Virginia Boyrevain's mother, Mrs. Kent, came back in August and honestly that poor woman. I wish I could tell you all she told us last night. Gin [Virginia] *and her baby are in Biarritz (occupied territory). Her husband, Jacque is in Paris, running his factory under Nazi eyes and Mrs. Kent has been arranging for Gin*

*and Danny (the little girl's about 3 years old) to return.
The boat passage is $375 for Gin and $175 for Danny,
$20 port tax at Lisbon and $10 cabling charge. She paid
the entire passage to Wash. DC and the gov't brings them
back or rather it's all arranged from one gov't to another.
So far she hasn't heard any news as to what's what for
when. Jacque had, I'm pretty sure, deposited most of his
wealth here, so Mrs. Kent doesn't want for anything. But,
oh she's so different from when I knew her in Paris! She's
seen so much suffering and now having her daughter over
there—golly I feel so sorry for her.*

*Incidentally, in a round about fashion I've some bad
news of Jacques Charles. He & Sandrini produced the Int'l
Casino show and he was producer at Paramount in Paris,
got me into Folies Bergère in Paris and was a* wonderful
*man and a fine friend of mine. He was Jewish. He was put
into a concentration camp (according to reports) and* died *of*
starvation*! It just makes me ill. I hope the report is wrong.
I'll let you know as I hear, about Gin & her little girl &
her husband. I think her husband is just biding his time or
else he's manufacturing phony ammunition.* I know him!

Reconnecting with friends from the French period in her
career was not always sad, though.

Friday aft., March 28 [just after her 30th
birthday]

*...Thanks a million for the birthday packages. I just
loved everything. ...WHO do you think walked in on me
last night and surprised me right out of my shoes!! Do you
remember Mary Brooks who was my roommate in Paris
when we were at the Paramount? I haven't seen her since*

Aug. 1933 when she left Biarritz to come home!! Well, did we ever have news for each other! She's out of show business now and working for her aunt & uncle in the advertising business. She saw the show from down in front about a month ago and recognized me!

Just saw Judy Garland in the elevator. She was leaving from her orchestra rehearsal for the benefit tonight. Sure is CUTE.

And more news from France.

Saturday night, Mar 29

…Had another letter from Roger today. He has an uncle in South America who has a job for him. Now, getting proper papers for his trip he says he can probably leave in a couple of months! He's going to try to come via New York. Wouldn't that be wonderful? Says he never wants a vacation for the rest of his life, he wants so much to work*!*

Her show business career now in its tenth year, Peg was just as close to her family as always. Her two younger sisters, Betty and Mary, were both working and still living at home. They made frequent visits to New York. Peg's older sister Ruth, had gone West in 1938 to get married. Her husband was an Army Captain. stationed at Ft. Huachuca, Arizona. Ruth was anxious to have her family come for a visit.

Friday night, April 11

…Ruth's letter sure is a peach. Sorry I've neglected returning it before. Gee, but it must be beautiful out there. Hope I can make it on my summer vacation (in the fall!)

...Haven't heard a word from Harry in 2 weeks! I'm not upset about it however, just amused. He probably thinks I'm eating my heart out!

Easter Sunday, April 13

...You know every year they have a Sunrise Service here at the Music Hall on Easter morning from 7-8. It's conducted by the NY Federation of Churches & is a non-sectarian service. I wanted to go to church, but how I hate mobs, so I decided to come here. I got up at 6 and was over here at 20 minutes to 7. You have never seen such droves and droves of people coming from every direction & by all means. They poured out of the subway constantly. Cabs lined up like mad in front constantly letting more people out—private cars, people walking from all streets and everyone pouring into the Music Hall. I stood in front & just watched until 5 to 7, then I came in and got a nice single seat in the first mezzanine. But it was jammed right up through the 3rd mezzanine and there were hundreds standing. This place seats around 6500! The service was lovely. The cathedral scene we use for the Easter pageant was on stage and there were, I don't know how many choristers, on stage. It sure was nice.

Roger continued to be able to get mail out of France. He was Peg's pipeline to all she had known and loved in that country.

Thursday, April 17

...Yesterday I had another letter from Roger. His kid brother, who has been missing since June last year, and about whom they've received smatterings of second &

fourth-hand news, is in Durban, So. Africa. They just found out!!

The young radio officer Peg had met on her way to South America in 1936, Charlie Stewart, was still a regular presence in her life. He was frequently in New York between sailings and they enjoyed spending time together.

Tuesday night, May 20

Your letter came this AM asking about whether I can come home this vacation. I'm off tomorrow night but I don't think I can make it. First of all, as much as I dislike having Charlie around for that long, I feel like it'd be sort of mean. He's so looking forward to having a week here. Of course I won't see him every day, but I can come home on my June vacation & he probably won't get the same opportunity again. And I sort of feel like even though it's a big bore to me, he's done so many especially nice things for me, that I should try my best to give him a few happy times. He expects so little & is so happy with his little.

Had a letter from Ruth too. She sent me snaps of her & of Van. He looks like he's lost weight, but he sure does look nice in his uniform. His anticipated maneuvers from Aug to Oct sure does put the blink on Mary's and my vacation trip. But then, from the looks of things Van will probably be fighting the war by that time. The way everyone speaks around here, sounds as if we'll be in it before June is out. I can't imagine it. I just can't believe that we'll be going through a "war"! It sort of scares me a little.

Wednesday night, June 4

...a notice from the US Treasury Dept announcing

my next installment due on my income tax!!! Us filthy
rich—ha ha—Honestly, I'm embarrassed when I make out
a money order for $7.07 income tax quarterly!!!…

The longer she was in show business, the more of a
perfectionist Peg became. Giving anything less than a perfect
performance was abhorrent to her.

Saturday night, June 28

I'm lower than a snake's belly right now & even
though I just mailed a letter home tonight, I just have to
write you again. The last show I made a terrible mistake
in line-up. It was the first step after the entrance (we enter
in line-up). Carol can't count the entrance so on the last
combination I've been saying "This is the last one." I got
myself used to saying different things like that during
rehearsals because I'm not used to "talking" a routine.
The girls around me know what they're doing. Well, after
the first show today, Carol asked me if I could say "kick
and down" on the last kick of the entrance, instead of the
way I had been saying it, because the way I was telling
her confused her. (Too G.D. bad about her!) So, the 2nd
and 3rd shows I said "kick and down" & this last show
I said it and was so darned busy thinking how to say it
I didn't know what the heck came next. So, I didn't do a
side kick and an inside fan kick, but got into it from there
on. I saw all these legs come up & didn't know what in the
world they were doing! Well, I've decided that Carol can
go plum to Hell as far as I'm concerned. I'm not going to
say another word in that number except counting the exit
which is OK. That doesn't upset me. But I'm just going to
be selfish enough to look out for myself from now on. Emily
didn't see my mistake. That doesn't matter. Whether she

saw it or not, I know I made it and I know it's not right. I still feel lousy. In fact I cried my eyes out about it & I know that's silly. But somehow when I do a thing like that, it takes away a bit of confidence. What infuriates me is that I wasn't even nervous opening show but the more we do it & the more mistakes Carol makes (& she does make plenty), the more I get scared. Of course, that's perfectly stupid & I'll put a stop to that starting the first show tomorrow!!

The nice opportunities still outnumbered the disappointments, by far.

Tuesday eve., July 1

...Russell [Markert, the choreographer] *called a bunch of us down to his office today & I was among them. At first I was sort of worried, and then I thought better of it. Turned out that 10 of us will do the "Minnie" (Rumba) a week from Wed. or Thurs. at that place in the Plaza where they skate or dance according to the season. Coty is opening a new place in Rockefeller Center and this is for the official opening. In return, we each will receive a beautiful leather make-up kit, filled with everything under the sun, and a bottle of L'Aimant as large as this piece of stationery! Nice, eh? It'll be at around 5:30, so it'll cut into our dinner hour, but so what! I think it'll be fun.*

...Charlie gets in next Mon. and that starts his vacation, 2 trips off. So when my week off comes, I'll go up to Taunton and meet his niece.

But Charlie was not the only name in Peg's date book.

Sunday aft., July 13

...The man I went out with Thursday night is a

Hollander. It was a blind date. Well, he is about the most interesting man I've ever met. He is 30 years old, but looks more like 35. Two hours after Holland fell, he left for England in a fishing boat & made it. He is in diplomatic service in London now & is head of the Code Dept. In the last year or so, he has gone around the world *I think, 4 times, by clipper most of the way. What a brilliant fellow! Not conceited either. And can he ever dance beautifully!*

He's here waiting for a Clipper for Lisbon. Hope he has to wait a while. He expects to be here at least another week, some mix-up on a visa. He has a diplomatic service passport & they won't give him a Portuguese visa except on a plain ordinary passport. So, he has to wait for that. Too many diplomats in Lisbon as it is, they say.

Saturday, July 19

…My friend I liked so much left Mon. for Wash. DC, for he didn't know how long, but he's supposed to come back to NY before going back to England—via a bomber from Halifax!!! I sure have the best luck of anyone I know!

Tuesday night, July 22

…My friend from Holland, or should I say from London, was sent from Wash DC to Canada & couldn't even take time to come to NY and he's taking a bomber back to England. I had a message from his cousin last night. Well, maybe it's just as well—but he was such a lot of fun.

In July, Charlie flew Peg up to Massachusetts to meet and spend some time with his family. The flight from LaGuardia to Boston was still quite a novelty. A one-way fare was $21.50 on American Airlines. While there, she took another crack at golf.

Monday night, July 28

...Fri. & Sat. we played golf. Thurs night we went out in the field in back of Shirley's (Charlie's niece) and practiced, so I was in a little better form Fri. AM. Of course, I can't even say I got a score, but I kept track just for fun. The course is 9-holes. For an 18-hole game par is usually around 90 or 85 I think. So, if you get 100 or even 105 you play a fairly decent game. Well, my score for 9 holes was a fairly decent score for 18! Fri. It was 109! Sat. I cut it down to 106! I wouldn't tell anyone but you folks & Virginia. But I got, accidentally I'm sure, 4 wonderful drives. The best was 146 yds. Charlie measured it off because it was such a nice one. And, at least I did connect. I got off from the first tee-off while 3 strange men were looking. That's such a nerve-wracking thing, and where I usually swing and miss about 4 times before I finally connect and tap the ball for about 25 yards! At any rate, I was quite pleased about the whole thing and could see marked improvement. Once I got in to a sand-trap and I took 7 shots to get out besides having the better part of the sand in my hair, ears, & mouth! Finally, I got good & mad & I got it out!

Peg's trip to Arizona with her sister, Mary, was still pending.

Wednesday, Aug 6

...Today I had a grand letter from Ruth & she says I should come on out there & we'll wait there for Mary.

She planned a 3-week vacation so was trying to take care of business before she left.

Friday, Aug 22

...Here's Daddy's money order for Sept on account of I won't be getting any salary in Sept, so better now than never, eh? I won't come back to work till Oct 9 and I have to wait a week before I'll get a check. I'm sending in my Sept. income tax payment today too. Getting stuff off my chest.

...Haven't started to pack a thing yet. Guess I'll take a couple of summer dresses for daytime in Arizona, and fall clothes. Will probably take my reversible for a coat & a pair of slacks and my suit. This is for Mary's information.

Peg left New York by train. She traveled through Chicago and Amarillo, arriving in Bisbee, Arizona, on September 12. Mary joined her a few days later. Not wanting Peg to be bored after the excitement of show business and life in New York, Ruth and Van arranged for Peg to meet a young Captain in Van's regiment. The tall, handsome, Earl Macherey, "Mac," a West Point graduate, swept Peg off her feet. They spent every possible moment together until she left with her sisters, Ruth and Mary, as planned, to drive to Bozeman, Montana, so the sisters from the East could meet Van's family. From Bozeman, the three planned to drive on to Cleveland.

Monday noon, Sept. 22 Bozeman, MT

...Now, first of all, please don't be disappointed, but Ruth & Mary will go to Cleveland without me. I've an extra week off and I'm going back to the Army! The way I figure is that I can get home very easily on my week off,

but I sure can't get out to Arizona in that time and since I was asked back & it was OK by everyone concerned , or not concerned, I'm going. Mac is such a peach of a fellow and we get along so well together, we just have to see a little more of each other. Had a wire from him this morning & he said if I could get my extra week, we'd go to a football game in Los Angeles on Oct 3! Mom, he's such a wonderful fellow. I couldn't even begin to compare him to anyone *I've* ever *known. And I'm not exaggerating or just having a flighty flirtation!*

Our trip up here was grand. Honestly, the beautiful wonders of our country are so much more than one can even imagine. We took loads of pictures around the Grand Canyon & I hope they are good. The only thing is that there was so much haze and I don't have a haze filter.

We're going into town this aft. And do a bit of shopping then we're going visiting, to a ranch (a farm in our language). It rained and snowed *between Salt Lake City & here, but it cleared up yesterday & is* beautiful *now.*

Oh gee folks, we are so happy—me especially. This is such a glorious vacation. I'm sure sorry we haven't written more, but I've been up to my neck having such a good time. In fact, Mac & I were on the go every evening & never got in before the wee hours.

A few days later, Peg and her sisters parted company. Ruth and Mary drove East to Cleveland and Peg took the train back to Arizona. On September 29, Peg cables her family in Cleveland.

Van and Mac met me at El Paso Mac and I were engaged between Las Cruses and Deming New Mexico

Will probably be married Thursday at Yuma if Mac can get leave From there probably drive to Los Angeles Letter follows Will wire from Yuma love from us both Peggy

True to her word, she filled the family in on the details later that same day.

Monday, Sept. 29 Ft. Huachuca

...I left here not knowing anything except that we were pretty crazy about each other, and that if at all possible, I was to come back after Bozeman.

Well, I left Laramie Sat. morning, changed trains in Denver, changed again in Dalhart, Texas at 9:30 PM and arrived in El Paso, Sunday at 8:30 AM. I was to change trains there also for Bisbee Junction. As I stepped off the train, I heard a red-cap say, "paging Miss Morrison" & I almost collapsed. He told me I was not to get on my next train, there was someone in the station waiting for me! Well, I was so excited I could hardly get to the station fast enough and as I was hurrying up the platform Mac met me! I can hardly remember anything from then on for a few minutes, except that the world was just we two, not another person existed on that crowded platform. Van was further up the way & we found him, and it was a glorious homecoming. They had decided at 8 or a little before, on Sat. night, to come to El Paso to meet me, left about 20 minutes later and drove 300 miles thru cloud bursts—arriving at 3 AM. We drove through more cloud bursts going back too, navigating flooded roads and dips and water like I have never before seen.

We left El Paso at about 10 AM, had lunch along the road around 11:30, when Van took the wheel. Mac said he'd gotten something at Sears Roebuck & did I want to see it! I couldn't imagine. Well, he opened the glove compartment & brought out a small (Tiffany's) box. It looked very much like it couldn't be anything but a ring. He took my left hand, the 3rd finger, opened up the box & put a ring on. It's the West Point ring, in a girl's size, just like the large man's type that he wears. It is natural yellow gold, with a light garnet in it, and has US emblems, etc, plus 1933—his year—on the side. It is really beautiful and I'd much rather have that instead of a diamond. Well, I swear, I don't know how I lived through such excitement. Mom, you'll love him & be so proud of him. I don't know how I can be so lucky, but I am. Van was excited too—golly I think he was as bad as Mac and I were.

We have not yet set the date. In fact, I haven't decided yet what kind of a wedding it will be. There are 3 choices, a large one on the Post (Ft. Huachuca), a small intimate one on the Post, or going away quietly to Yuma or someplace like that & then send out announcements right away instead of invitations for the other. For my part, I'd like the last of the 3, but I feel that is selfish. Naturally, I'm a little scared of all the Army life, I know nothing about it, and yet this Army life is Mac's life and will be mine. So, I feel that for his sake we should have it on the Post. I definitely couldn't think of a large wedding, I guess I wasn't built for that, but I could go through a small one all right. Anyhow, it's still in the near future and plenty of time to decide.

Now, about my job. Don't you ever worry about me not giving sufficient notice. I am writing airmail this morning to Russell and since I have to go to NY anyhow,

I'll be there when I was supposed to & if he wants me to "work out a notice" I will. Otherwise, I'll just do all the things I have to do and come back here. For one thing, I have to get my income tax figured for this present year and pay that. There is so much to do there like that—round up all my junk—I'm sure I'll have to get another trunk, get my coat out of storage, and of course, see Charlie & tell him all about it. That's something else, Mom, I'll certainly do my best to tell him so he won't be hurt. I know that Charlie has been waiting for this to happen ever since he met me, so it won't be too great a shock. I'll try my very best—Charlie is worth the "best" for all his faithfulness & kindnesses. I know that alright.

We are trying to get up a party for the LA trip, Van & another fellow, and we 2 of course. That will fill the car, and be a nice crowd for the jaunt, and I'll be perfectly chaperoned. As a matter of fact Mom, you need never worry about Mac's morals. He is as fine as they come, Mom, and again I say, I surely am a lucky girl.

I'll close now. Sure hope Ruth & Mary are both fine and stood the trip OK.

PS Mac just came over & we've decided to go to Yuma on Wed and get married quietly there. Of course, we will wire you right away as soon as it happens. He says he prefers it that way & so do I. I'm so happy I can't concentrate on a thing. Hardly even know my own name. Please, please don't worry about this step. I know just as sure as you're my Mom that Mac & I are for each other.

And so, the storybook career had a storybook ending. Peg and Mac were married in Yuma, Arizona, on October

2. They honeymooned in Los Angeles. Then Peg returned to New York, arriving October 8, to work out her notice. When she walked into rehearsal the next day showing off her ring, Russell Markert responded, "So, you go off on vacation and come back engaged." Peg remembered, "I showed him the two rings and said, 'I'll have you know there are four days between those two rings!'" Over the next three weeks, she tied up the loose ends of one life and prepared to enter another. As Peg hung up her ballet and tap shoes, she closed the book on a remarkable odyssey.

She arrived back in Arizona on November 4, 1941, to begin her new career...Army Wife Extraordinaire. Peggy Morrison, now Mrs. Earl J. Macherey, entered her new life with the same passion, enthusiasm and commitment she had taken to New York ten years earlier.

EPILOGUE

Life as an Army Wife fed Peg's wanderlust. and her gregarious personality. She and Mac served several tours in Central and South America where her Spanish fluency was a real asset. As the wife of the Military Attaché, she was frequently called upon to perform official social duties, a role she executed with ease and grace.

Peg reflects on her post-Rockette life.

"Becoming Mac's wife, my life went from GREAT to GREATER. Our first home was in Bisbee, Arizona. It was there that we experienced Pearl Harbor Day. From that time on, it was a succession of fascinating assignments and travels.

"Mac served in General Douglas MacArthur's Headquarters in Brisbane, Australia during the war. The children and I accompanied him on all his post-war assignments Some of the highlights included, Quito, Ecuador, here he was Chief of the US Military Mission; San Salvador, El Salvador where he again served as Chief of the US Military Mission.

"While we were stationed in El Salvador Mac had his one and only opportunity to se me dance. I was asked to put on a dance for an amateur theatrical group. I selected 10 or 12 women and choreographed their number. The final night of their performance, one of the gals feigned illness so I would have to replace her and Mac would get to see me dance!

"Our last overseas assignment was in Montevideo, Uruguay where Mac was US Army Military Attaché. President

Eisenhower came for an official visit while we were there. Vice President and Mrs. Nixon had come to El Salvador during our tour of duty there. Those kinds of festivities were part of our life as members of the 'official delegation' in foreign countries. My life was very exciting, so I never really missed the 'glitz and glamour' of show business."

Today this remarkable woman, now 90-plus years young, lives in Nashville, Tennessee and says, "I've truly had a fantastic life and at age 92 am one happy person!" She lives with her daughter, Carol, a partner in a veterinary hospital there. Peg works out daily, manages the household, runs the errands and cares for their menagerie (four dogs and a cat). Her son, Doug, lives with his family in the Washington, DC area. Her granddaughter, Laura, is a junior at Virginia Tech.

What of the cast of characters? Most of them have passed on…Mac; the matchmakers, Ruth and Van; and all of the women with whom she roomed over the years. When she told Charlie Stewart about her marriage, he said he would not contact her again, "It just wouldn't be right." Roger Sasso, her French friend, came through New York after the war on his way to Rio in 1946. Unable to contact Peg, he sent a lengthy letter to her parents, detailing his wartime work for the French Resistance and the post-war emotional demise of their mutual friend, René.

Only a few Rockettes from Peg's time are still living. But Thursday night generally finds Peg at her computer, typing away on the Rockettes' chat line. She is definitely still connected to that prestigious sorority she joined in 1939.

***

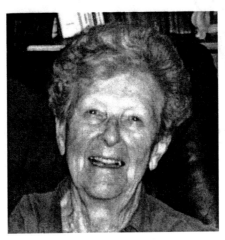

Peg on her 90th

***

Peggy Morrison Macherey celebrated her 90th birthday in March of 2001, surrounded by her children and granddaughter. They sipped Piper Heidsiek champagne, her favorite ever since the 1932 voyage to France. A white stretch limousine whisked them off to an elegant dinner at the Wild Boar in Nashville. Flowers were sent from all over the country, but perhaps the best bouquet of all came from the Rockette Alumni Association.

In August 2001, she joined other Rockette alumnae in New York to celebrate the Rockettes 75th Anniversary. The highlight of the week, was a dance, performed by several current Rockettes and all able-bodied alumnae. Peggy Morrison Macherey was the oldest dancer that day on 6th Ave in front of Radio City Music Hall. She loved every second of it!

***

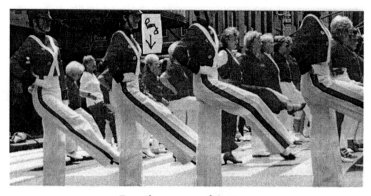

Peg dances on 6th Ave.
Rockette's 75th Anniversary Celebration

***

Peg was indeed fortunate to be part of the entertainment industry in its golden era. She was truly a participant in history. She retired her dancing shoes just one month before Pearl Harbor. The entertainment industry she had known, like so many other things, would be forever changed.

ACKNOWLEDGEMENTS

My father, too, was a career Army Officer. However, we were always stationed a world apart from the Machereys, so we only saw them once every four or five years. I grew up knowing that my Aunt Peg had been a Rockette, but the actual scope of her show business carrer was a mystery to me until that fateful day in 1995 when she first captivated my husband. So, this has been a journey of discovery for me and I'm indebted to many people who made it possible.

First and foremost, my maternal grandmother, Florence Morrison, who had the foresight to save all those letters. The gaps occur largely because she shared some of the more extraordinary letters with others who were negligent in returning them. After my grandmother died, my Aunt Betty preserved the treasure. Without the diligence of these two women, most of the stories and experiences would be lost.

And secondly, to my late mother, Ruth Morrison Van Fleet, who forfeited her scholarship and college education in 1930 to return home and share financial responsibility for the family. Her willingness to assume this responsibility freed Peg to pursue her dreams.

Peg's recall is amazing, but the day to day experiences that make the story real are only possible through letters. I believe all three of the sisters enjoyed their involvement in this project. Especially helpful were Betty's remembrances of New York in

1934 and Mary's recollections of their life on Taylor Road in Cleveland.

Additionally, to my husband, Dave, who first recognized the value in preserving Peg's experiences. His remark, "I sure hope someone is writing this stuff down" became my call to action. He has encouraged and supported me every step of the way.

And finally, to the dear friends and family who helped by proofing and re-proofing, most notably, my sister and brother-in-law, Rae & Lloyd Marquis and my dear friend Grace Bettison, the comma queen.

I've always known my parents left me an interesting and unusual legacy. Discovering this dimension of that legacy is a gift I'll treasure forever.

Ro Trent Vaselaar
September 2003

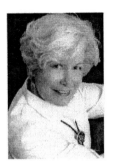

R o Trent Vaselaar grew up an Army brat and has lived all over the world.

Retired from a career in travel and tourism, she lives now in Anthem, Arizona, with her husband, Dave and their Westie, Sushi.

The niece of Peg Macherey, Vaselaar began this project as a way to preserve the stories for her family, but quickly realized that it was a story worth sharing.